Color Atlas of

LARGE ANIMAL APPLIED ANATOMY

Hilary M Clayton
BVMS PhD MRCVS
Professor of Veterinary Anatomy
Western College of Veterinary Medicine
University of Saskatchewan
Saskatoon, Saskatchewan
Canada

Peter F Flood
BVSc MSc PhD MRCVS
Professor of Veterinary Anatomy
Western College of Veterinary Medicine
University of Saskatchewan
Saskatoon, Saskatchewan
Canada

with

David Mandeville
ABIPP
Division of Audio Visual Services
University of Saskatchewan
Saskatoon, Saskatchewan
Canada

Charles Farrow
DVM Dip ACVR
Professor of Veterinary Anesthesiology, Radiology and Surgery
Western College of Veterinary Medicine
Saskatoon, Saskatchewan
Canada

Mosby-Wolfe

London Baltimore Bogotá Boston Buenos Aires Caracas Carlsbad, CA Chicago Madrid Mexico City Milan Naples, FL New York Philadelphia St. Louis Sydney Tokyo Toronto Wiesbaden

Published in 1996 by Mosby-Wolfe, an imprint of Times Mirror International Publishers Limited.

Printed by Grafos, S.A. arte sobre papel, Barcelona, Spain.

ISBN 0 7234 1717 2

For full details of all Times Mirror International Publishers Limited titles, please write to Times Mirror International Publishers Limited, Lynton House, 7–12 Tavistock Square, London WC1H 9LB, England.

A CIP catalogue record for this book is available from the British Library.

Library of Congress Cataloging-in-Publication Data applied for.

Project Manager:	Peter Harrison
Designer	Rob Curran
Layout Artist:	Lindy van den Berghe
Cover Design:	Paul Phillips
Production:	Siobhan Egan
Index:	Anita Reid
Publisher:	Jane Hunter

Contents

Acknowledgements

Mr Bob Famulak spent uncounted hours dissecting specimens and assembling skeletal material. We recognize the quality of his work and appreciate his meticulous attention to detail. The contributions of Dr Olin Balch, Dr. Karen Timm and Ms Glenna Miller in securing suitable specimens and the anatomical preparations are gratefully acknowledged.

Last, but certainly not least, we thank Mrs Carol Ross who typed the bulk of the manuscript and cheerfully keyed in the numerous revisions.

1 Introduction

This atlas contains anatomical photographs of five large domestic herbivores, the horse (*Equus caballus*), the ox (*Bos taurus*), the sheep (*Ovis aries*), the llama (*Lama glama*) and the pig (*Sus scrofa*). It is not intended to be a substitute for a conventional anatomical reference book, of which there are several; instead it is an illuminating companion to the texts for those starting on their anatomical studies and a source of insight and specialized information for the more advanced reader.

Modern photographic and colour printing techniques have been exploited to provide the most realistic images possible of prepared bones and rapidly dissected, unfixed tissues, giving detailed conceptual information that cannot be readily obtained by other means. Some structures, such as the abdominal viscera, deteriorate rapidly in the fresh state and in these cases we have given high priority to the accurate portrayal of colour and texture, and been content with relatively simple dissections.

The study of anatomy takes as its subject the form and relationships of the parts of bodies. Communication between anatomists is facilitated by the use of agreed standardized terms and a list of these has been developed and periodically revised by the International Committee on Veterinary Anatomical Nomenclature. The list, which forms a small book, is known as the Nomina Anatomica Veterinaria (NAV)[1] and it provides general descriptive terms applicable to all vertebrates, and specific terms related to the structure of the domestic animals. During the preparation of the NAV, every effort has been made to maximize conformity between the human and domestic animal nomenclatures but because veterinary terminology must be based on the normal quadrupedal stance rather than the erect human position, there are distinct differences in the terms used for direction. The veterinary terms are related to parts of the body, thus blood that flows towards the head is said to flow cranially and that which flows towards the tail flows caudally. The directional terms are described in detail in this introduction using annotated photographs of a horse.

Whenever possible, each anatomical concept is defined in Latin in the NAV by a short, simple term with instructive and descriptive value. Anatomists are encouraged to translate the original Latin terms into their own languages unless this leads to obvious ambiguity. In general, anglicized terms have been used in this Atlas, although the Latin terms have been retained for muscles. When a structure has a synonym or well-known name in common usage, it is shown in brackets.

Unfortunately the NAV is not yet universal and it does not, for example, provide detailed terms for the stomach of the llama. Thus for this structure our terminology was derived from that used by Vallenas *et al.*[2]

1. *Nomina Anatomica Veterinaria* (1983, 3rd edition). International Committee on Veterinary Gross Anatomical Nomenclature, Ithaca, New York.

2. Vallenas, A., Cummings, J.F. and Munnell, J.F. (1971). A gross study of the compartmentalized stomach of two New World camelids, the llama and guanaco, *Journal of Morphology*, **134**, 399–424.

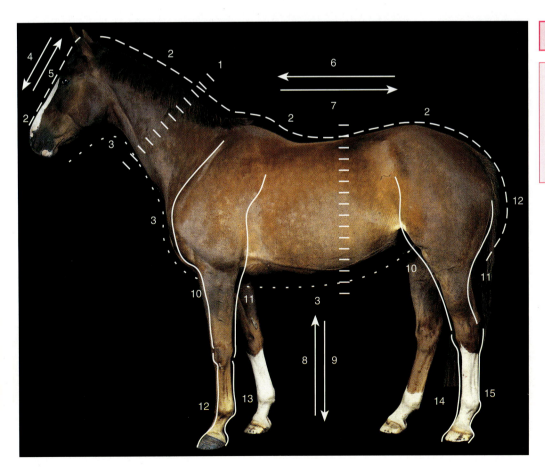

1. Live horse, lateral view. Topographical terms.

1 Transverse plane – neck, trunk	7 Caudal – neck, trunk, tail
2 Dorsal – head, neck, trunk, tail	8 Proximal – limb
	9 Distal – limb
3 Ventral – head, neck, trunk, tail	10 Cranial – proximal limb
	11 Caudal – proximal limb
4 Rostral – head	12 Dorsal – manus
5 Caudal – head	13 Palmar – manus
6 Cranial – neck, trunk, tail	14 Dorsal – pes
	15 Plantar – pes

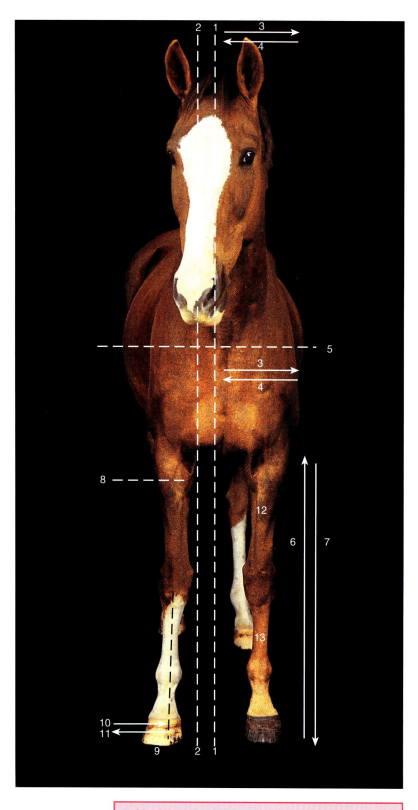

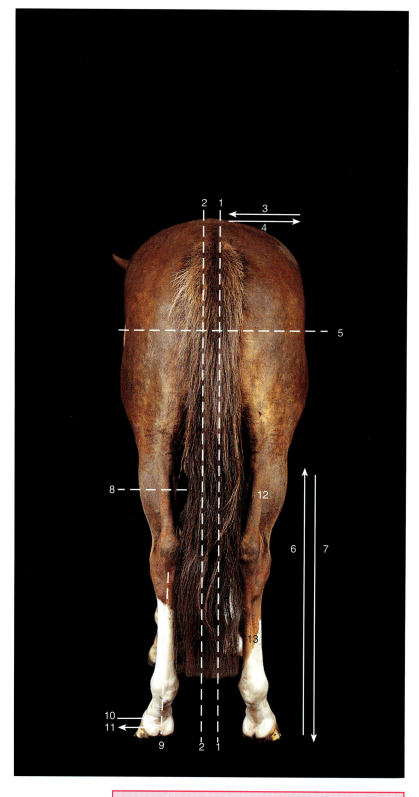

2. Live horse, frontal view. Topographical terms.

3. Live horse, caudal view. Topographical terms.

Head, neck, trunk	Limbs
1 Median plane	6 Proximal
2 Sagittal plane	7 Distal
3 Lateral	8 Transverse plane
4 Medial	9 Axial plane
5 Dorsal plane	10 Axial
	11 Abaxial
	12 Cranial
	13 Dorsal

Head, neck, trunk	Limbs
1 Median plane	6 Proximal
2 Sagittal plane	7 Distal
3 Lateral	8 Transverse plane
4 Medial	9 Axial plane
5 Dorsal plane	10 Axial
	11 Abaxial
	12 Caudal
	13 Plantar

2 Head

In this chapter palpable landmarks are indicated on photographs of live animals, osteological features are shown on bone specimens, and soft tissue structures are revealed using a series of prepared dissections. Topographical relationships between the bones and soft tissue structures are clarified, using specimens that have been sectioned in various orientations, and radiographs.

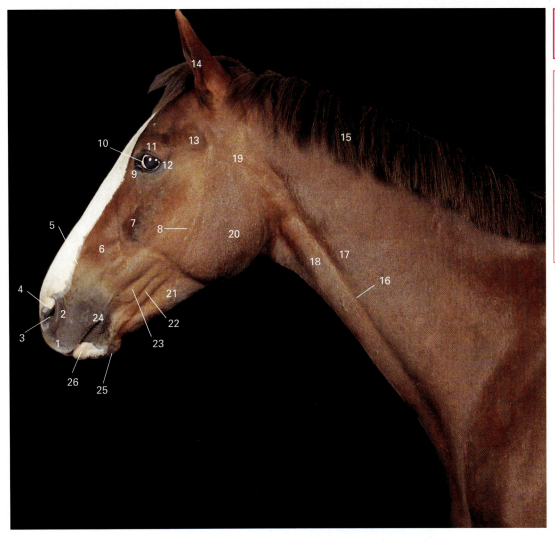

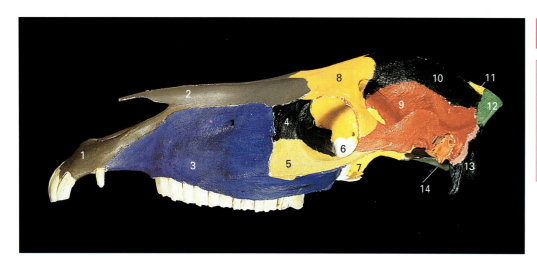

5. Bones of skull of horse, lateral view.

1 Incisive bone	9 Temporal bone
2 Nasal bone	10 Parietal bone
3 Maxilla	11 Interparietal bone
4 Lacrimal bone	12 Occipital bone,
5 Zygomatic bone	squamous part
6 Palatine bone,	13 Occipital bone, lateral
perpendicular plate	part
7 Presphenoid bone	14 Occipital bone, basilar
8 Frontal bone	part

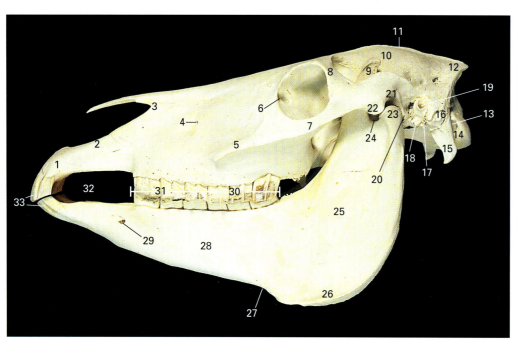
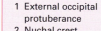

6. Skull and mandible of female horse, lateral view.

1 Body of incisive bone	17 Stylomastoid foramen
2 Nasal process of incisive	18 Styloid process
bone	19 External acoustic meatus
3 Nasoincisive notch	20 Retroarticular process
4 Infraorbital foramen	21 Mandibular fossa
5 Facial crest	22 Articular tubercle
6 Fossa for lacrimal sac	23 Condylar process
7 Zygomatic arch	24 Mandibular notch
8 Zygomatic process of	25 Ramus of mandible
frontal bone	26 Angle of mandible
9 Coronoid process	27 Notch for facial vessels
10 Temporal fossa	28 Body of mandible
11 External sagittal crest	29 Mental foramen
12 Nuchal crest	30 Molar teeth
13 Condyloid fossa	31 Premolar teeth
14 Occipital condyle	32 Interalveolar border
15 Paracondylar process	33 Incisor teeth
16 Mastoid process	

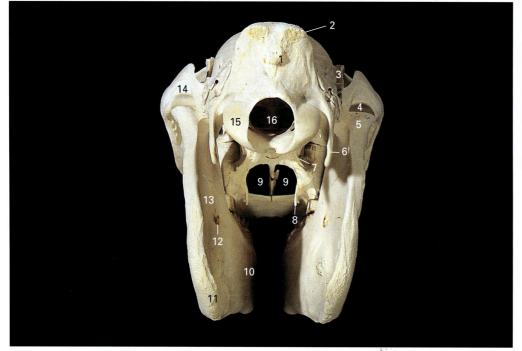

7. Skull and mandible of horse, caudal view.

1 External occipital	9 Choanae
protuberance	10 Body of mandible
2 Nuchal crest	11 Angle of mandible
3 Coronoid process	12 Mandibular foramen
4 Mandibular fossa	13 Ramus of mandible
5 Condylar process	14 Zygomatic arch
6 Paracondylar process	15 Occipital condyle
7 Caudal alar foramen	16 Foramen magnum
8 Hamulus of pterygoid	

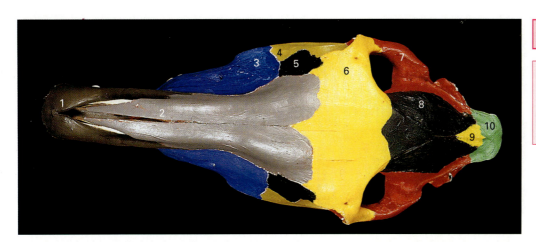

8. Bones of skull of horse, dorsal view.

1 Incisive bone	7 Temporal bone
2 Nasal bone	8 Parietal bone
3 Maxilla	9 Interparietal bone
4 Zygomatic bone	10 Occipital bone,
5 Lacrimal bone	squamous part
6 Frontal bone	

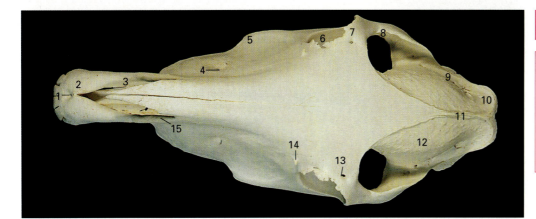

9. Skull of horse, dorsal view.

1 Interincisive canal	8 Zygomatic arch
2 Body of incisive bone	9 Temporal line
3 Nasal process of incisive	10 Nuchal crest
bone	11 External sagittal crest
4 Infraorbital foramen	12 Temporal fossa
5 Facial crest	13 Supraorbital foramen
6 Orbit	14 Rostral lacrimal process
7 Zygomatic process of	15 Nasoincisive notch
frontal bone	

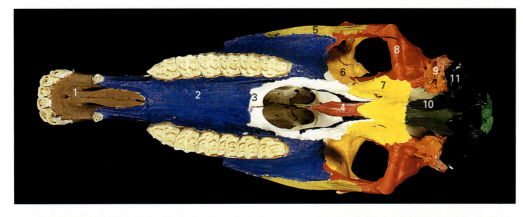

10. Bones of skull of horse, ventral view.

1 Incisive bone	8 Temporal bone, squamous
2 Maxilla	part
3 Palatine bone	9 Temporal bone, tympanic
4 Vomer	and petrous parts
5 Zygomatic bone	10 Occipital bone, basilar
6 Frontal bone	part
7 Sphenoid bone	11 Occipital bone, lateral
	part

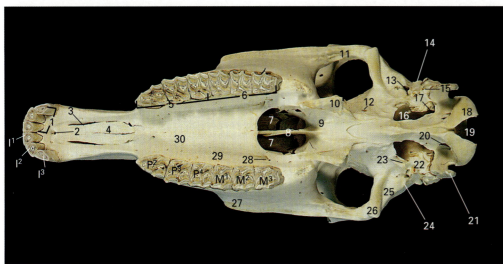

11. Skull of female horse, ventral view.

1 Incisor teeth (I^1, I^2, I^3)	16 Foramen lacerum
2 Interincisive canal	17 Jugular foramen
3 Palatine fissure	18 Occipital condyle
4 Palatine process of incisive	19 Foramen magnum
bone	20 Hypoglossal canal
5 Premolar teeth (P^2, P^3, P^4)	21 Paracondylar process
6 Molar teeth (M^1, M^2, M^3)	22 Tympanic bulla
7 Choanae	23 Osseous part of auditory
8 Vomer	tube
9 Wings of vomer	24 Retroarticular process
10 Hamulus of pterygoid	25 Mandibular fossa
bone	26 Articular tubercle
11 Zygomatic arch	27 Rostral end of facial crest
12 Caudal alar foramen	28 Major palatine foramen
13 Petrotympanic fissure	29 Palatine groove
14 External acoustic meatus	30 Palatine process of
15 Stylomastoid foramen	maxilla

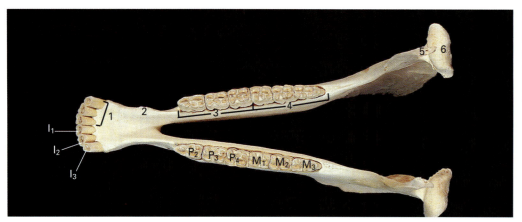

12. Mandible of female horse, dorsal view.

1 Incisor teeth (I_1, I_2, I_3)	4 Molar teeth (M_1, M_2, M_3)
2 Interalveolar border	5 Coronoid process
3 Premolar teeth (P_2, P_3, P_4)	6 Condylar process

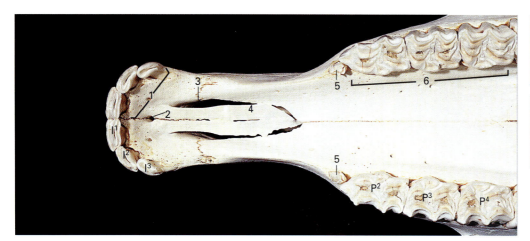

13. Rostral part of skull of female horse, ventral view, showing the position of the first premolar (wolf) tooth, which is sometimes present in horses of either sex.

1 Incisor teeth (I^1, I^2, I^3)	5 First upper premolar
2 Interincisive canal	(wolf) tooth (P^1)
3 Palatine fissure	6 Premolar teeth (P^2, P^3, P^4)
4 Palatine process of incisive bone	

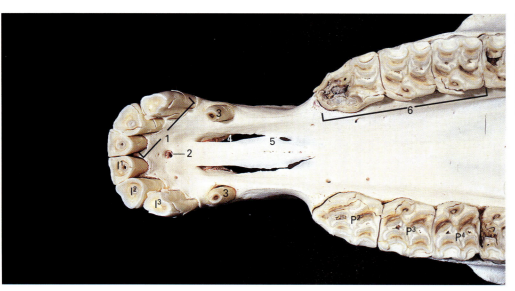

14. Rostral part of skull of male horse, ventral view.

1 Incisor teeth (I^1, I^2, I^3)	5 Palatine process
2 Interincisive canal	6 Premolar teeth
3 Canine tooth	(P^2, P^3, P^4)
4 Palatine fissure	

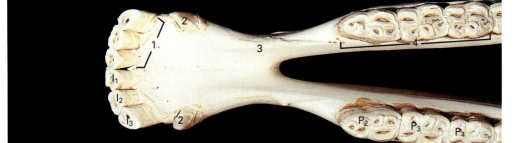

15. Rostral part of mandible of male horse, dorsal view.

1 Incisor teeth (I_1, I_2, I_3)	4 Premolar teeth
2 Canine tooth	(P_2, P_3, P_4)
3 Interalveolar border	

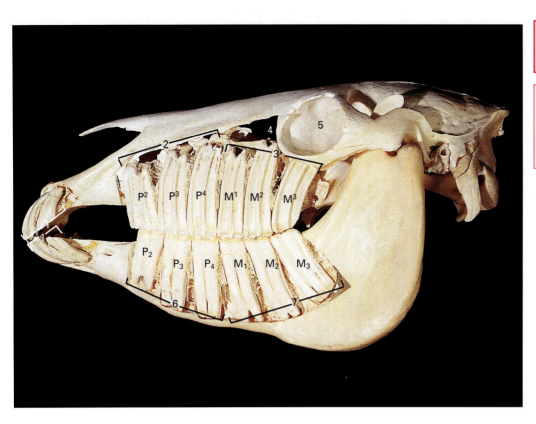

16. Skull of young adult horse, lateral view. The bones have been sculptured to show the extent of the reserve crowns of the incisors, premolars and molars.

1 Incisor teeth	5 Orbit
2 Upper premolar teeth (P^2, P^3, P^4)	6 Lower premolar teeth (P_2, P_3, P_4)
3 Upper molar teeth (M^1, M^2, M^3)	7 Lower molar teeth (M_1, M_2, M_3)
4 Maxillary sinus	

- Deciduous dentition of horse:

$$2\{Di\ ^3/_3;\ Dp\ ^3/_3\}$$

- Permanent dentition of horse:

Male $2\{I\ ^3/_3;\ C\ ^1/_1;\ P\ ^{3\ or\ 4}/_3;\ M\ ^3/_3\}$

Female $2\{I\ ^3/_3;\ C\ ^0/_0;\ P\ ^{3\ or\ 4}/_3;\ M\ ^3/_3\}$

- The second, third and fourth premolars are consistently present in the upper and lower jaws. The first upper premolar is vestigial or absent in both sexes. When present it forms part of the permanent dentition.

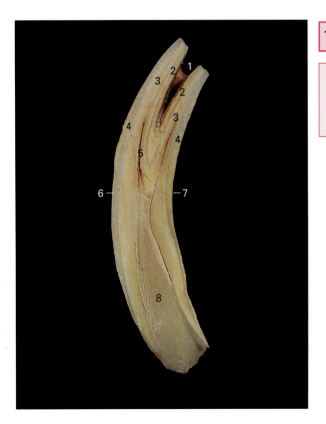

17. Incisor tooth of young horse, longitudinal section.

1 Infundibulum	5 Secondary dentin will appear as the dental star
2 Central enamel	6 Rostral (buccal) surface
3 Dentin	7 Caudal (lingual) surface
4 Peripheral enamel	8 Pulp cavity

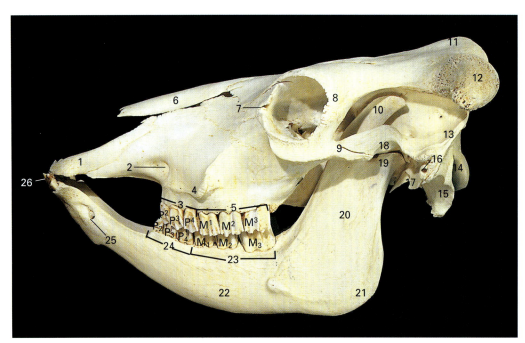

18. Skull and mandible of ox, lateral view.

1 Incisive bone	14 Occipital condyle
2 Infraorbital foramen	15 Paracondylar process
3 Upper premolar teeth (P^2,	16 External acoustic meatus
P^3, P^4)	17 Tympanic bulla
4 Facial tuber	18 Articular tubercle
5 Upper molar teeth (M^1, M^2,	19 Condylar process
M^3)	20 Ramus of mandible
6 Nasal bone	21 Angle of mandible
7 Fossa for lacrimal sac	22 Body of mandible
8 Zygomatic process	23 Lower molar teeth
9 Zygomatic arch	(M_1, M_2, M_3)
10 Coronoid process	24 Lower premolar teeth
11 Intercornual protuberance	(P_2, P_3, P_4)
12 Cornual process	25 Mental foramen
13 Temporal line	26 Lower incisor and canine
	teeth

- Deciduous dentition of ox:

$$2 \{ Di\ ^0/_3;\ Dc\ ^0/_1;\ Dp\ ^3/_3 \}$$

- Permanent dentition of ox:

$$2 \{ I\ ^0/_3;\ C\ ^0/_1;\ P\ ^3/_3;\ M\ ^3/_3 \}$$

- The lower canine tooth is situated lateral and adjacent to the third incisor, and it resembles an incisor tooth in size and shape.
- The first premolar is absent in the upper and lower arcades.

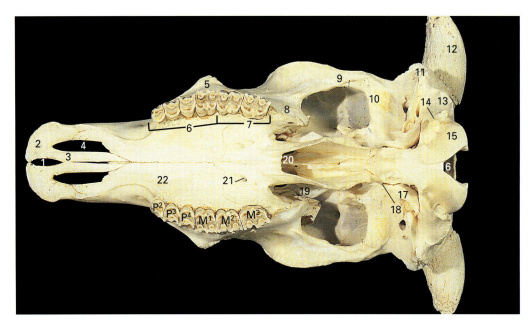

19. Skull of ox, ventral view.

1 Interincisive fissure	12 Cornual process
2 Body of incisive bone	13 Paracondylar process
3 Palatine process of incisive	14 Hypoglossal canal
bone	15 Occipital condyle
4 Palatine fissure	16 Foramen magnum
5 Facial tuber	17 Tympanic bulla
6 Upper premolar teeth	18 Oval foramen
(P^2, P^3, P^4)	19 Hamulus of pterygoid
7 Upper molar teeth	bone
(M^1, M^2, M^3)	20 Choanae
8 Maxillary tuber	21 Major palatine foramen
9 Zygomatic arch	22 Palatine process of
10 Articular tubercle	maxilla
11 External acoustic meatus	

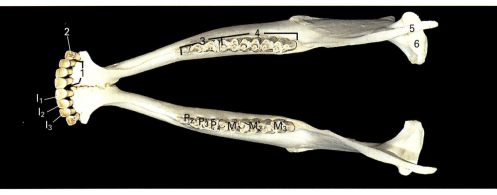

20. Mandible of ox, dorsal view.

1 Lower incisor teeth	4 Lower molar teeth
(I_1, I_2, I_3)	(M_1, M_2, M_3)
2 Canine tooth	5 Coronoid process
3 Lower premolar teeth	6 Condylar process
(P_2, P_3, P_4)	

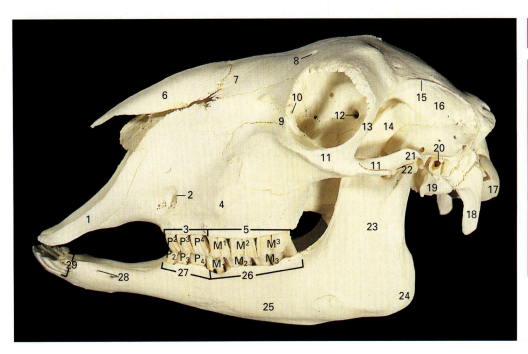

21. Skull and mandible of sheep, lateral view.

1	Incisive bone	16	Temporal fossa
2	Infraorbital foramen	17	Occipital condyle
3	Upper premolar teeth (P^2, P^3, P^4)	18	Paracondylar process
4	Facial tuber	19	Tympanic bulla
5	Upper molar teeth (M^1, M^2, M^3)	20	External acoustic meatus
6	Nasal bone	21	Articular tubercle
7	Frontal bone	22	Condylar process
8	Supraorbital foramen	23	Ramus of mandible
9	External lacrimal fossa	24	Angle of mandible
10	Fossa for lacrimal sac	25	Body of mandible
11	Zygomatic arch	26	Lower molar teeth (M_1, M_2, M_3)
12	Optic canal	27	Lower premolar teeth (P_2, P_3, P_4)
13	Zygomatic process	28	Mental foramina
14	Coronoid process	29	Lower incisor and canine teeth
15	Temporal line		

- Deciduous dentition of sheep:
$$2 \{ Di \ ^0/_3; \ Dc \ ^0/_1; \ Dp \ ^3/_3 \}$$
- Permanent dentition of sheep:
$$2 \{ I \ ^0/_3; \ C \ ^0/_1; \ P \ ^3/_3; \ M \ ^3/_3 \}$$

- The lower canine tooth is situated lateral and adjacent to the third incisor, and it resembles an incisor tooth in size and shape.
- The first premolar is absent in the upper and lower arcades.

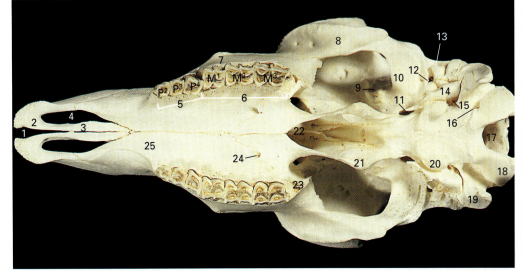

22. Skull of sheep, ventral view.

1	Interincisive fissure	12	External opening of temporal meatus
2	Body of incisive bone	13	External acoustic meatus
3	Palatine process of incisive bone	14	Tympanic bulla
4	Palatine fissure	15	Jugular foramen
5	Upper premolar teeth (P^2, P^3, P^4)	16	Hypoglossal canal
6	Upper molar teeth (M^1, M^2, M^3)	17	Foramen magnum
7	Facial tuber	18	Occipital condyle
8	Zygomatic arch	19	Paracondylar process
9	Orbital opening of supraorbital canal	20	Muscular tubercle
10	Articular tubercle	21	Hamulus of pterygoid bone
11	Oval foramen	22	Choanae
		23	Maxillary tuber
		24	Major palatine foramen
		25	Palatine process of maxilla

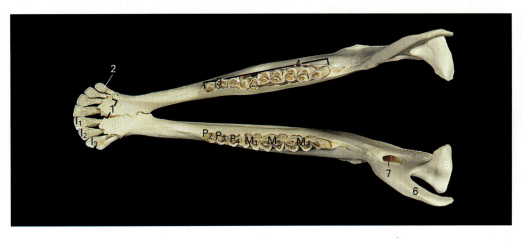

23. Mandible of sheep, dorsal view.

1	Lower incisor teeth (I_1, I_2, I_3)	4	Lower molar teeth (M_1, M_2, M_3)
2	Lower canine tooth	5	Condylar process
3	Lower premolar teeth (P_2, P_3, P_4)	6	Coronoid process
		7	Mandibular foramen

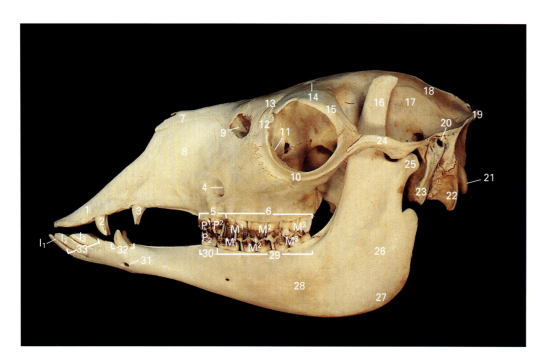

24. Skull and mandible of llama, lateral view.

1 Incisive bone	18 Parietal bone
2 Upper incisor tooth	19 Nuchal crest
3 Upper canine tooth	20 External acoustic meatus
4 Infraorbital foramen	21 Occipital condyle
5 Upper premolar teeth (P^1, P^2)	22 Paracondylar process
6 Upper molar teeth (M^1, M^2, M^3)	23 Tympanic bulla
	24 Zygomatic arch
7 Nasal bone	25 Condylar process
8 Maxilla	26 Ramus of mandible
9 Nasolacrimal fissure	27 Angle of mandible
10 Zygomatic bone	28 Body of mandible
11 Nasolacrimal canal	29 Lower molar teeth (M_1, M_2, M_3)
12 Lacrimal bone	
13 Frontal bone	30 Lower premolar tooth (P_2)
14 Supraorbital foramen	31 Mental foramen
15 Supraorbital process	32 Lower canine tooth
16 Coronoid process	33 Lower incisor teeth (I_1, I_2, I_3)
17 Temporal bone	

- Deciduous dentition of llama:

$$2 \{ Di\ ^1/_3;\ Dp\ ^{2-3}/_{1-2} \}$$

- Permanent dentition of llama:

$$2 \{ I\ ^1/_3;\ C\ ^1/_1;\ P\ ^{1-2}/_{1-2};\ M\ ^3/_3 \}$$

- Deciduous canine teeth are occasionally present in males, but rarely erupt in females.
- Eruption of permanent canine teeth is variable in females and castrated males.
- The upper incisor is caniniform.

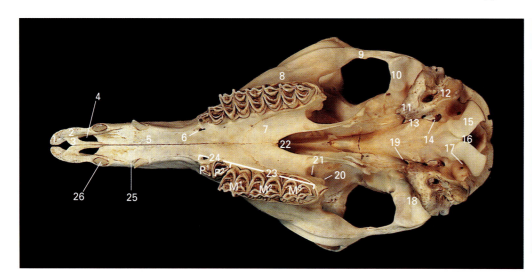

25. Skull of llama, ventral view.

1 Body of incisive bone	14 Jugular foramen
2 Nasal process of incisive bone	15 Occipital condyle
	16 Foramen magnum
3 Palatine process of incisive bone	17 Hypoglossal canal
	18 Retroarticular process
4 Palatine fissure	19 Oval foramen
5 Palatine process of maxilla	20 Supraorbital canal
6 Major palatine foramen	21 Sphenopalatine foramen
7 Palatine bone	22 Choanae
8 Zygomatic bone	23 Upper molar teeth (M^1, M^2, M^3)
9 Zygomatic arch	
10 Articular tubercle	24 Upper premolar teeth (P^1, P^2)
11 Tympanic bulla	
12 Paracondylar process	25 Upper canine tooth
13 Muscular tubercle	26 Upper incisor tooth

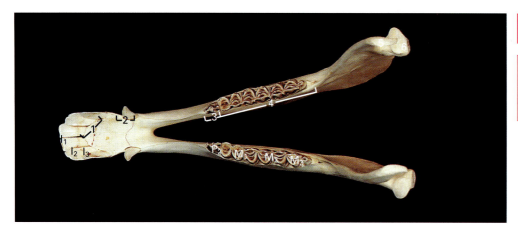

26. Mandible of llama, dorsal view.

1 Lower incisor teeth (I_1, I_2, I_3)	4 Lower molar teeth (M_1, M_2, M_3)
2 Lower canine tooth	5 Coronoid process
3 Lower premolar tooth (P_2)	6 Condylar process

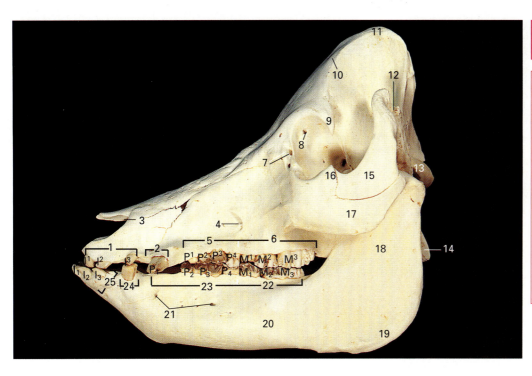

27. Skull and mandible of pig, lateral view. The rostral bone is not shown.

1 Upper incisor teeth (I¹, I², I³)	14 Paracondylar process
2 Upper canine tooth	15 Zygomatic process of temporal bone
3 Nasoincisive notch	16 Frontal process of zygomatic bone
4 Infraorbital foramen	17 Temporal process of zygomatic bone
5 Upper premolar teeth (P¹, P², P³, P⁴)	18 Ramus of mandible
6 Upper molar teeth (M¹, M², M³)	19 Angle of mandible
7 Lacrimal foramina	20 Body of mandible
8 Orbital opening of supraorbital canal	21 Mental foramina
9 Zygomatic process of frontal bone	22 Lower molar teeth (M₁, M₂, M₃)
10 Temporal line	23 Lower premolar teeth (P₁, P₂, P₃, P₄)
11 Nuchal crest	24 Lower canine tooth
12 External acoustic meatus	25 Lower incisor teeth (I₁, I₂, I₃)
13 Occipital condyle	

- Deciduous dentition of pig:

$$2 \{Di\ ^3/_3;\ Dc\ ^1/_1;\ Dp\ ^3/_3\}$$

- Permanent dentition of pig:

$$2 \{I\ ^3/_3;\ C\ ^1/_1;\ P\ ^4/_4;\ M\ ^3/_3\}$$

- The canine teeth (tushes) are better developed in the males.

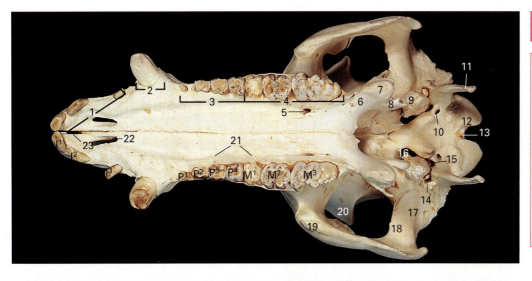

28. Skull of pig, ventral view.

1 Upper incisor teeth (I¹, I², I³)	11 Paracondylar process
2 Upper canine tooth	12 Occipital condyle
3 Upper premolar teeth (P¹, P², P³, P⁴)	13 Intercondylar incisure
4 Upper molar teeth (M¹, M², M³)	14 Stylomastoid foramen
5 Major palatine foramen	15 Jugular foramen
6 Palatine bone	16 Foramen lacerum
7 Pyramidal process of palatine bone	17 Mandibular fossa
8 Hamulus of pterygoid bone	18 Articular tubercle
9 Tympanic bulla	19 Zygomatic arch
10 Hypoglossal canal	20 Zygomatic process of frontal bone
	21 Palatine groove
	22 Palatine fissure
	23 Interincisive fissure

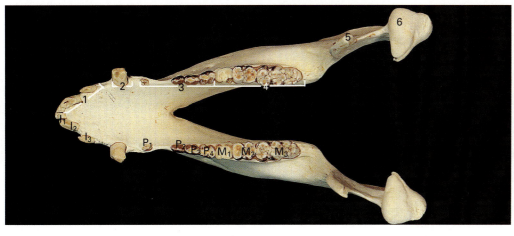

29. Mandible of pig, dorsal view.

1 Lower incisor teeth (I₁, I₂, I₃)	4 Lower molar teeth (M₁, M₂, M₃)
2 Lower canine tooth	5 Coronoid process
3 Lower premolar teeth (P₁, P₂, P₃, P₄)	6 Condylar process

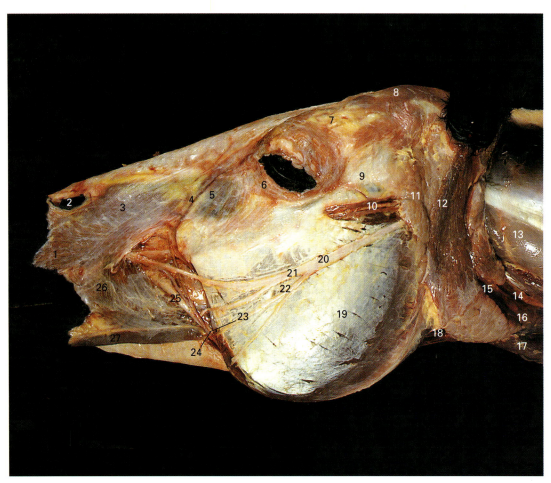

30. Superficial dissection of head of horse, lateral view. Cutaneous muscles have been removed.

1 M. caninus	15 Maxillary vein
2 Nasal diverticulum	16 External jugular vein
3 M. levator nasolabialis	17 M. sternocephalicus
4 Angular vein of eye	18 M. sternohyoideus
5 M. levator labii	19 M. masseter
superioris	20 Facial nerve (VII)
6 M. orbicularis oculi	21 Dorsal buccal branch
7 Supraorbital fat pad	of facial nerve
8 M. temporalis	22 Ventral buccal branch
9 Zygomatic arch	of facial nerve
10 Transverse facial	23 Facial vein
vessels	24 Facial artery
11 Parotid gland	25 Parotid duct
12 M. parotidoauricularis	26 M. buccinator
13 M. brachiocephalicus	27 M. depressor labii
14 Common carotid artery	inferioris

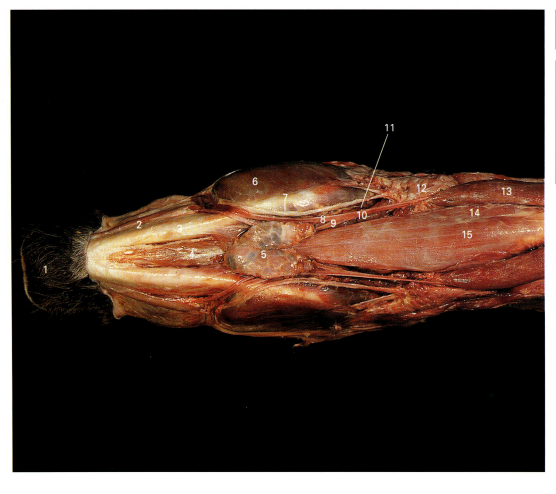

31. Superficial dissection of head of horse, ventral view. Cutaneous muscles have been removed.

1 Chin	8 Facial vein
2 M. depressor labii	9 Lingual vein
inferioris	10 Linguofacial vein
3 Mandible	11 Facial artery
4 M. mylohyoideus	12 Parotid gland
5 Mandibular lymph	13 M. sternocephalicus
node	14 M. omohyoideus
6 M. masseter	15 M. sternohyoideus
7 Parotid duct	

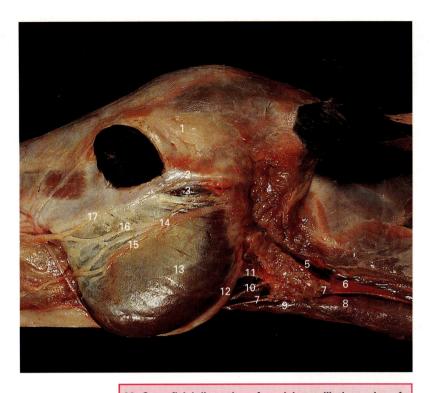

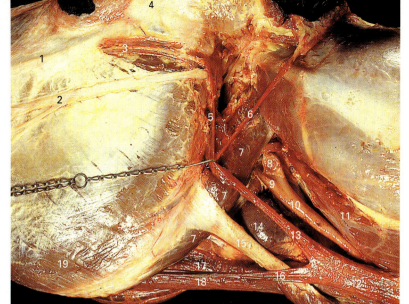

32. Superficial dissection of caudal mandibular region of horse, lateral view. Cutaneous muscles and M. parotidoauricularis have been removed.

1 Supraorbital fat pad
2 Zygomatic arch
3 Transverse facial vessels
4 Parotid gland
5 Maxillary vein
6 External jugular vein
7 Linguofacial vein
8 M. sternocephalicus
9 M. sternohyoideus and M. omohyoideus
10 Parotid duct
11 Tendon of M. sternocephalicus
12 Edge of mandible
13 M. masseter
14 Facial nerve (VII)
15 Ventral buccal branch of facial nerve
16 Dorsal buccal branch of facial nerve
17 Facial crest

33. Deep dissection of caudal mandibular region of horse, ventrolateral view. The M. parotidoauricularis, the parotid gland and the mandibular gland have been removed. The maxillary vein has been retracted rostrally.

1 Facial crest
2 Buccal branch of facial nerve
3 Transverse facial vessels and nerve
4 Zygomatic arch
5 Superficial temporal vein
6 Caudal auricular vein
7 M. digastricus
8 Carotid sinus on internal carotid artery
9 External carotid artery
10 Common carotid artery
11 M. omotransversarius
12 External jugular vein
13 Maxillary vein
14 Thyroid gland
15 Tendon of M. sternocephalicus
16 Linguofacial vein
17 M. sternothyroideus
18 M. sternohyoideus and M. omohyoideus
19 M. masseter

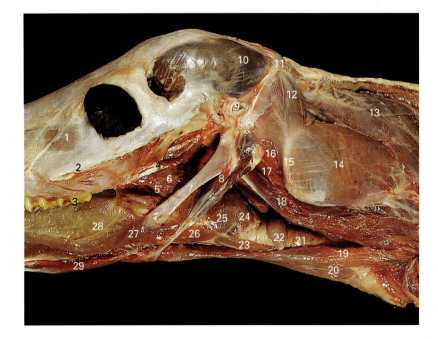

34. Deep dissection of caudal mandibular region of foal. Left mandible has been removed.

1 M. levator labii superioris
2 Facial crest
3 First upper molar tooth (M^1)
4 M. tensor veli palatini
5 M. palatopharyngeus
6 M. pterygopharyngeus
7 Stylohyoid bone
8 M. stylohyoideus
9 External auditory canal
10 M. temporalis
11 Nuchal crest
12 M. obliquus capitis cranialis
13 M. splenius
14 M. brachiocephalicus
15 Wing of atlas
16 M. rectus capitis lateralis
17 M. rectus capitis ventralis
18 M. longus capitis
19 M. omohyoideus
20 M. sternohyoideus
21 Trachea
22 Thyroid gland
23 M. sternothyroideus
24 M. cricopharyngeus
25 M. thyropharyngeus
26 M. thyrohyoideus
27 M. styloglossus
28 Tongue
29 M. geniohyoideus

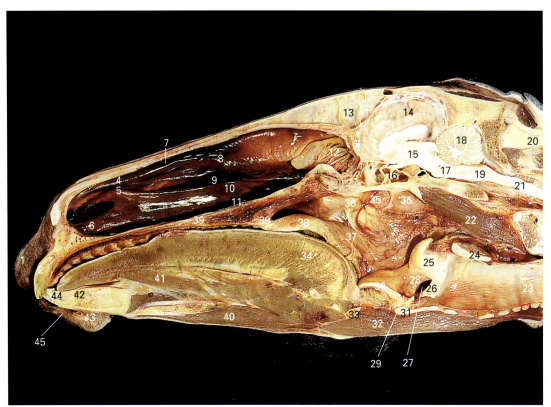

35. Paramedian section through head of horse. Nasal septum has been removed.

1	Upper lip	25	Arytenoid cartilage
2	Incisor tooth (I^1)	26	Vocal fold
3	Alar cartilage	27	Lateral laryngeal ventricle
4	Straight fold	28	Vestibular fold
5	Alar fold	29	Median laryngeal ventricle
6	Basal fold		
7	Dorsal meatus	30	Epiglottis
8	Dorsal nasal concha	31	Thyroid cartilage
9	Middle meatus	32	M. sternohyoideus
10	Ventral nasal concha	33	Basihyoid bone
11	Ventral meatus	34	M. genioglossus
12	Ethmoidal conchae	35	Mucosa separating left and right auditory tube diverticulae
13	Septum separating left and right frontal sinuses	36	Opening of auditory tube
14	Cerebral hemisphere	37	Nasopharynx
15	Cerebral crura	38	Soft palate
16	Sphenopalatine sinus	39	Hard palate
17	Pons	40	M. geniohyoideus
18	Cerebellum	41	M. styloglossus
19	Medulla oblongata	42	Mandible
20	Nuchal ligament	43	Chin
21	Spinal cord	44	Incisor tooth (I_1)
22	M. longus capitis	45	Lower lip
23	Trachea		
24	Cricoid cartilage		

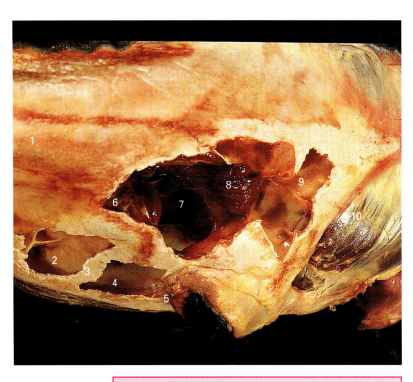

36. Dissection of frontal and maxillary region of head of horse, dorsal view. Overlying bone has been removed to expose the interior of the frontal and maxillary sinsuses.

1	Nasal bone	7	Frontomaxillary opening
2	Rostral maxillary sinus	8	Ethmoidal conchae in frontal sinus
3	Maxillary sinus septum	9	Frontal sinus
4	Caudal maxillary sinus	10	M. temporalis
5	M. orbicularis oculi		
6	Conchal part of frontal sinus		

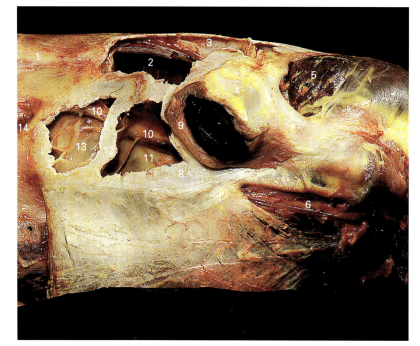

37. Dissection of frontal and maxillary region of head of horse, lateral view. Overlying bone has been removed to expose the interior of the frontal and maxillary sinuses.

1	Nasal bone	8	Facial crest
2	Conchal part of frontal sinus	9	M. orbicularis oculi
3	Frontal sinus	10	Infraorbital canal
4	Supraorbital fat pad	11	Caudal maxillary sinus
5	M. temporalis	12	Maxillary sinus septum
6	Transverse facial vessels	13	Rostral maxillary sinus
7	Zygomatic arch	14	Infraorbital foramen

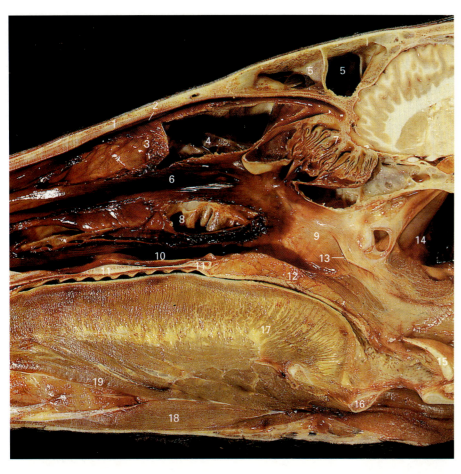

38. Paramedian section through head of horse. The medial walls of the dorsal and ventral conchae have been removed.

1 Nasal bone	10 Ventral meatus
2 Dorsal meatus	11 Hard palate
3 Scrolled portion of dorsal nasal concha	12 Soft palate
4 Conchal portion of frontal sinus	13 Opening of auditory tube
	14 Auditory tube diverticulum (guttural pouch)
5 Frontal sinus	15 Epiglottis
6 Middle meatus	16 Basihyoid bone
7 Ethmoidal conchae	17 Tongue
8 Conchal portion of rostral maxillary sinus	18 M. geniohyoideus
9 Nasopharynx	19 M. hyoglossus

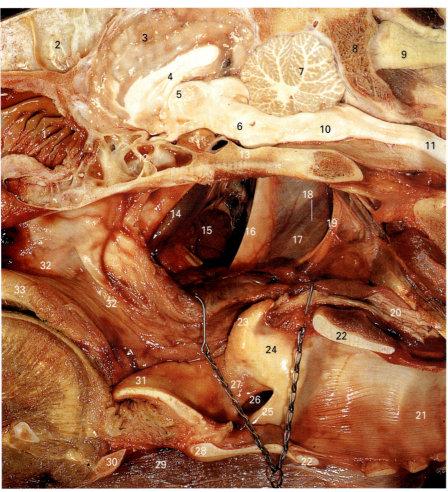

39. Paramedian section through pharynx and larynx of horse. The floor of the auditory tube diverticulum has been retracted ventrally to reveal its interior.

1 Ethmoidal conchae	17 Lateral compartment of auditory tube diverticulum
2 Midline septum between left and right frontal sinuses	18 Glossopharyngeal nerve (IX)
3 Cerebral hemisphere	19 Hypoglossal nerve (XII)
4 Corpus callosum	20 Oesophagus
5 Interthalamic adhesion	21 Trachea
6 Mesencephalon	22 Cricoid cartilage
7 Cerebellum	23 Corniculate process
8 Occipital bone	24 Arytenoid cartilage
9 Nuchal ligament	25 Vocal fold
10 Medulla oblongata	26 Lateral laryngeal ventricle
11 Spinal cord	27 Vestibular fold
12 Sphenoidal sinus	28 Thyroid cartilage
13 Basisphenoid and presphenoid bones	29 M. sternohyoideus and M. omohyoideus
14 Auditory tube	30 Basihyoid bone
15 Medial compartment of auditory tube diverticulum	31 Epiglottis
	32 Nasopharynx
16 Stylohyoid bone	33 Soft palate

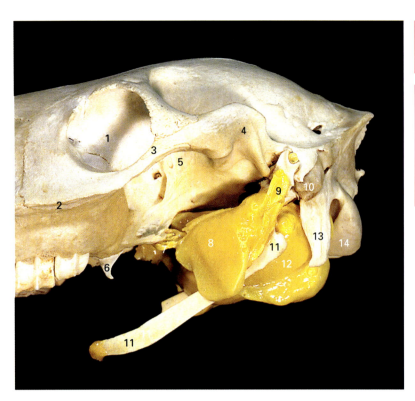

40. Skull of horse, lateral view. The external auditory canals, auditory tubes and auditory tube diverticulae (guttural pouches) have been filled with yellow latex.

1 Orbit	8 Lateral compartment of
2 Facial crest	auditory tube diverticulum
3 Zygomatic arch	9 External acoustic meatus
4 Mandibular fossa	10 Mastoid process
5 Pterygopalatine fossa	11 Stylohyoid bone
6 Hamulus of pterygoid	12 Medial compartment of
bone	auditory tube diverticulum
7 Auditory tube	13 Paracondylar process
	14 Occipital condyle

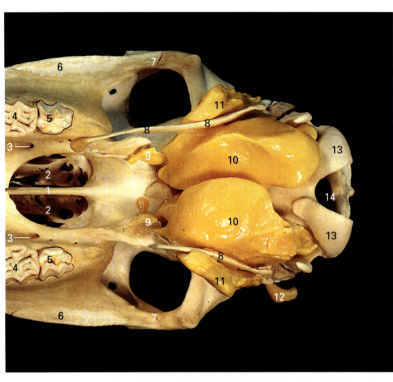

41. Skull of horse, ventral view. The external auditory canals, auditory tubes and auditory tube diverticulae (guttural pouches) have been filled with yellow latex.

1 Vomer	10 Medial compartment
2 Choanae	of auditory tube
3 Major palatine foramen	diverticulum
4 Second upper molar	11 Lateral compartment of
5 Third upper molar	auditory tube
6 Facial crest	diverticulum
7 Zygomatic arch	12 External auditory canal
8 Stylohyoid bone	13 Occipital condyle
9 Auditory tube	14 Foramen magnum

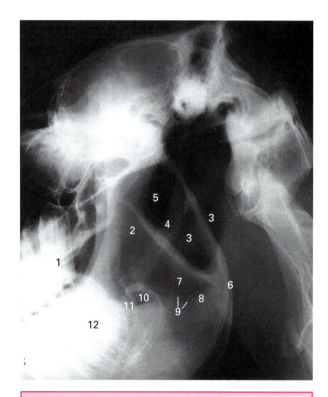

42. Radiograph of mandibular region of horse, lateromedial projection.

1 Upper third molar	7 Laryngopharynx
2 Nasopharynx	8 Corniculate process of
3 Medial compartment of	arytenoid cartilage
auditory tube diverticulum	9 Aryepiglottic folds
4 Stylohyoid bone	10 Epiglottis
5 Lateral compartment of	11 Soft palate
auditory tube diverticulum	12 Third lower molar
6 Edge of mandible	

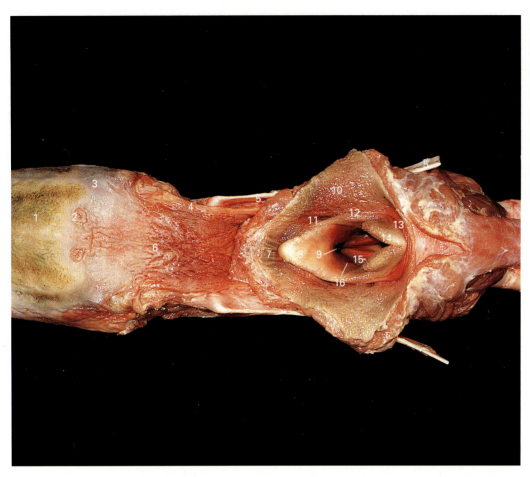

43. Tongue and larynx of horse. The aditus laryngis has been exposed by opening the pharynx dorsally.

1 Dorsum of tongue	10 Wall of pharynx
2 Vallate papilla	11 Piriform recess (lateral
3 Foliate papilla	food channel)
4 Palatoglossal fold	12 Aryepiglottic fold
5 Stylohyoid bone	13 Dorsal part of
6 Root of tongue	palatopharyngeal arch
7 Caudal extremity of soft	14 Corniculate process of
palate	arytenoid cartilage
8 Epiglottis	15 Vocal fold
9 Median ventricle of larynx	16 Lateral laryngeal ventricle

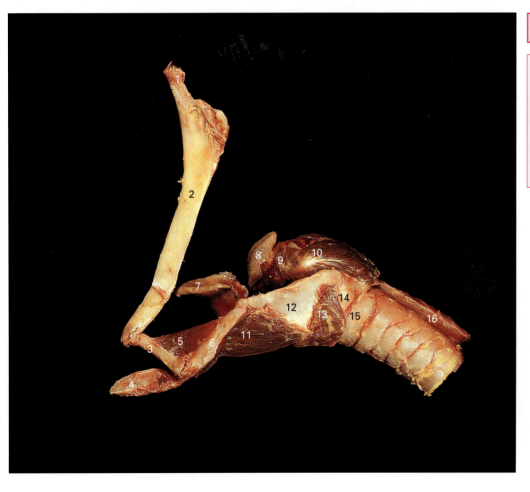

44. Larynx and hyoid bones of horse, lateral view.

1 Tympanohyoid bone	10 M. cricoarytenoideus
2 Stylohyoid bone	dorsalis
3 Ceratohyoid bone	11 M. thyrohyoideus
4 Lingual process	12 Thyroid cartilage
5 M. ceratohyoideus	13 M. cricothyroideus
6 Thyrohyoid bone	14 Cricoid cartilage
7 Epiglottis	15 First tracheal ring
8 Arytenoid cartilage	16 Oesophagus
9 M. arytenoideus	
transversus	

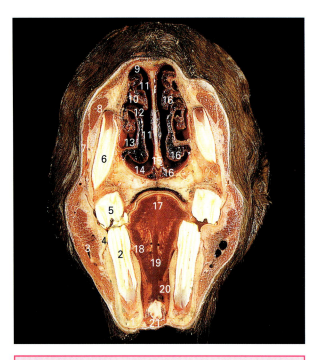

45. Transverse section through head of horse. Section is cut at the level of the third premolar tooth.

1 Mandible	11 Common nasal meatus
2 Third lower premolar	12 Middle nasal meatus
3 M. masseter	13 Ventral nasal concha
4 Buccal glands	14 Ventral nasal meatus
5 Third upper premolar	15 Nasal septum
6 Reserve crown and root of	16 Nasal venous plexus
second upper premolar	17 Body of tongue
7 M. levator nasolabialis	18 M. hyoglossus
8 M. levator labii superioris	19 M. genioglossus
9 Dorsal nasal meatus	20 Sublingual gland
10 Dorsal nasal concha	21 M. geniohyoideus

46. Transverse section through head of horse. Section is cut at the level of the third molar tooth.

1 Mandible	11 Conchal part of maxillary
2 M. masseter	sinus
3 Reserve crown and root of	12 Infraorbital canal
second lower molar	13 Nasal septum
4 Third lower molar	14 Hard palate
5 Third upper molar	15 Body of tongue
6 M. levator labii superioris	16 M. genioglossus
and M. levator nasolabialis	17 M. hyoglossus
7 Nasolacrimal duct	18 Mandibular duct
8 Conchofrontal sinus	19 Sublingual vessels
9 Rostral part of maxillary	20 M. geniohyoideus
sinus	21 M. mylohyoideus
10 Caudal part of maxillary	
sinus	

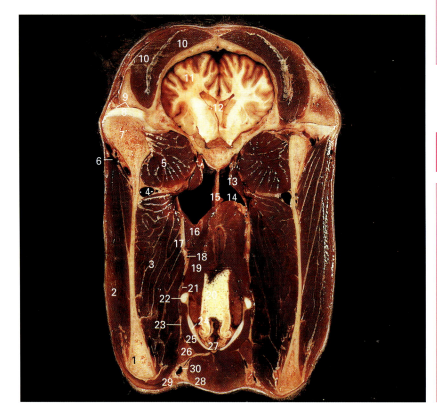

47. Transverse section through head of horse. Section is cut at the level of the temporomandibular joint.

1 Mandible	17 Stylohyoid bone
2 M. masseter	18 Lingual artery and nerve
3 M. pterygoideus medialis	19 M. hyopharyngeus
4 Maxillary vein	20 Epiglottis
5 M. pterygoideus lateralis	21 Facial artery
6 Transverse facial vessels	22 Rostral cornu of thyroid
7 Condylar process	cartilage
8 Articular disc	23 Tendon of M. digastricus
9 Mandibular fossa	24 Thyroid cartilage
10 M. temporalis	25 M. thyrohyoideus
11 Cerebral hemisphere	26 Mandibular gland
12 Lateral ventricle of brain	27 Median ventricle of
13 M. tensor veli palatini	larynx
14 Auditory tube diverticulum	28 M. omohyoideus and M.
(guttural pouch)	sternohyoideus
15 Midline septum	29 M. cutaneus fasciei
16 M. stylopharyngeus	30 Linguofacial vein

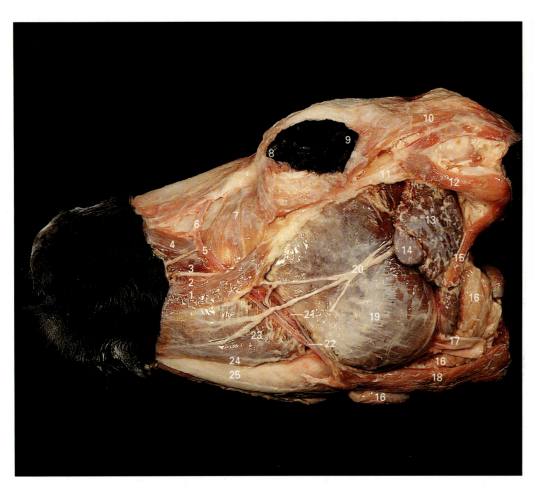

48. Superficial dissection of head of ox, lateral view. Cutaneous muscles have been removed.

1 M. zygomaticus	14 Parotid lymph node
2 M. depressor labii superioris	15 M. parotidoauricularis
3 M. caninus	16 Mandibular gland
4 M. levator labii superioris	17 External jugular vein
5 Facial vein	18 M. sternomandibularis
6 Angular vein of eye	19 M. masseter
7 M. malaris	20 Dorsal buccal branch of facial nerve
8 Medial commissure of eyelids	21 Parotid duct
9 Lateral commissure of eyelids	22 Facial vessels and ventral buccal branch of facial nerve
10 M. frontalis	23 M. buccinator
11 Zygomatic arch	24 M. depressor labii inferioris
12 M. zygomaticoauricularis	25 Body of mandible
13 Parotid gland	

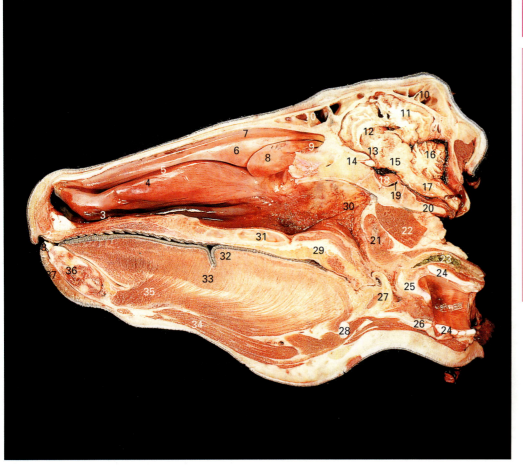

49. Paramedian section through head of ox. Nasal septum has been removed.

1 Upper lip	21 Medial retropharyngeal lymph node
2 Dental pad	22 M. longus capitis
3 Ventral nasal meatus	23 Oesophagus
4 Ventral nasal concha	24 Cricoid cartilage
5 Middle nasal meatus	25 Arytenoid cartilage
6 Dorsal nasal concha	26 Thyroid cartilage
7 Dorsal nasal meatus	27 Epiglottis
8 Middle nasal concha	28 Basihyoid bone
9 Ethmoidal conchae	29 Soft palate
10 Frontal sinus	30 Nasopharynx
11 Cerebral hemisphere	31 Palatine sinus
12 Lateral ventricle of brain	32 Torus linguae
13 Third ventricle of brain	33 Fossa linguae
14 Optic chiasma	34 M. geniohyoideus
15 Interthalamic adhesion	35 M. genioglossus
16 Cerebellum	36 Mandible
17 Medulla oblongata	37 Lower lip
18 Hypophysis	38 Lower incisor tooth
19 Cavernous sinus	
20 Occipital bone	

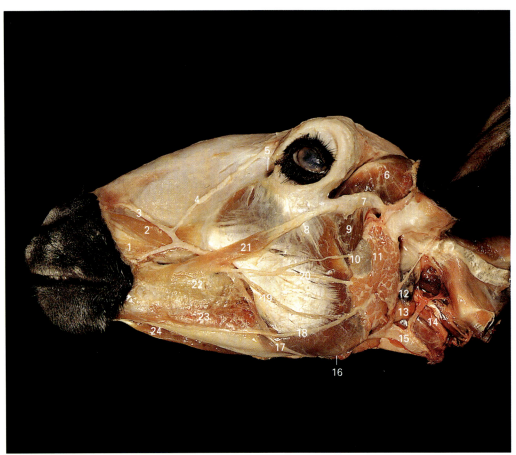

1 M. levator labii superioris	13 Mandibular gland
2 M. caninus	14 Common carotid artery
3 Dorsal nasal vein	15 External jugular vein
4 Angular vein of eye	16 Mandibular lymph node
5 Fossa for gland of infraorbital sinus	17 Facial vein
6 M. temporalis	18 Ventral buccal branch of facial nerve
7 Zygomatic arch	19 Parotid duct
8 M. masseter, superficial part	20 Dorsal buccal branch of facial nerve
9 M. masseter, deep part	21 M. zygomaticus
10 Parotid lymph node	22 M. buccinator
11 Parotid gland	23 M. depressor labii inferioris
12 Lateral retropharyngeal lymph node	24 M. mylohyoideus

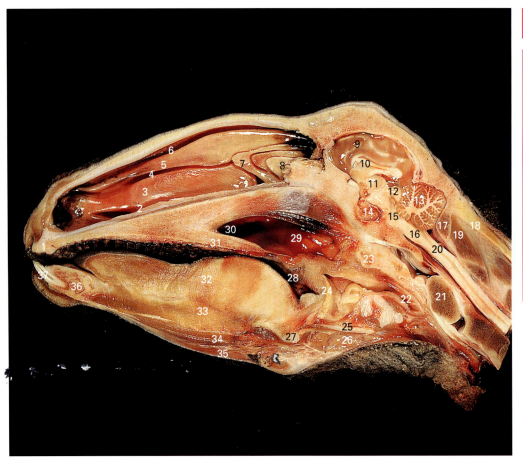

51. Paramedian section of head of sheep.

1 Dental pad	21 Atlas
2 Ventral nasal meatus	22 Oesophagus
3 Ventral nasal concha	23 Medial retropharyngeal lymph node
4 Middle nasal meatus	24 Epiglottis
5 Dorsal nasal concha	25 Thyroid cartilage
6 Dorsal nasal meatus	26 Mandibular gland
7 Middle nasal concha	27 Basihyoid bone
8 Ethmoidal conchae	28 Oropharynx
9 Cerebral hemisphere	29 Nasopharynx
10 Lateral ventricle of brain	30 Choana
11 Thalamus	31 Palatine process of maxilla (hard palate)
12 Rostral colliculus	32 Body of tongue
13 Cerebellum	33 M. genioglossus
14 Hypophysis	34 M. geniohyoideus
15 Pons	35 M. mylohyoideus
16 Medulla oblongata	36 Mandible
17 Occipital bone	37 Lower incisor
18 Nuchal ligament	
19 M. rectus capitis dorsalis	
20 Spinal cord	

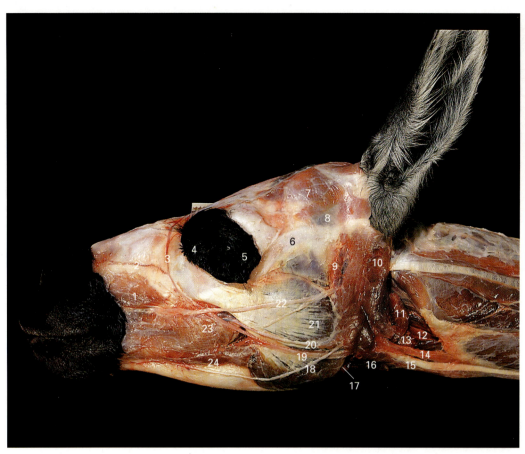

1	M. levator labii superioris	14	External jugular vein
2	Dorsal nasal vein	15	M. sternocephalicus
3	Angular vein of eye	16	M. sternohyoideus
4	Medial commissure of eyelids	17	Mandibular lymph nodes
5	Lateral commissure of eyelids	18	Ventral buccal branch of facial nerve
6	Zygomatic arch	19	Facial artery and vein
7	M. frontalis	20	Parotid duct
8	M. temporalis	21	M. masseter
9	Parotid lymph node	22	Dorsal buccal branch of facial nerve
10	Parotid gland	23	M. buccinator
11	Mandibular gland	24	M. depressor labii inferioris
12	Common carotid artery		
13	Lateral retropharyngeal lymph node		

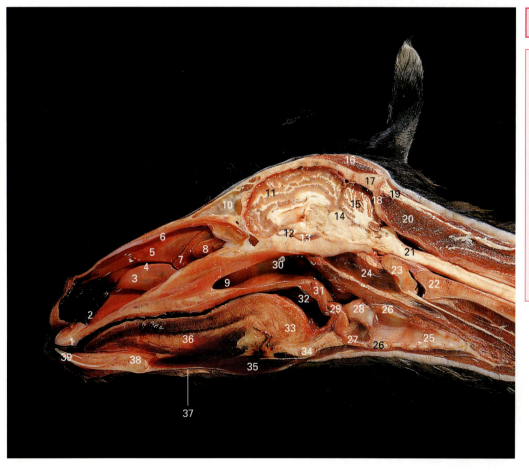

53. Paramedian section of head of llama.

1	Dental pad	20	M. semispinalis capitis
2	Ventral nasal meatus	21	Spinal cord
3	Ventral nasal concha	22	Axis
4	Middle nasal meatus	23	Atlas
5	Dorsal nasal concha	24	M. longus capitis
6	Dorsal nasal meatus	25	Trachea
7	Middle nasal concha	26	Cricoid cartilage
8	Ethmoidal conchae	27	Thyroid cartilage
9	Choana	28	Arytenoid cartilage
10	Frontal sinus	29	Epiglottis
11	Cerebral hemisphere	30	Nasopharynx
12	Optic chiasma	31	Soft palate
13	Hypophysis	32	Oropharynx
14	Rostral colliculus	33	Root of tongue
15	Cerebellum	34	Basihyoid bone
16	M. temporalis	35	M. geniohyoideus
17	Nuchal crest	36	M. genioglossus
18	Occipital bone	37	M. mylohyoideus
19	Funicular part of nuchal ligament	38	Mandible
		39	Lower incisor tooth (I_1)

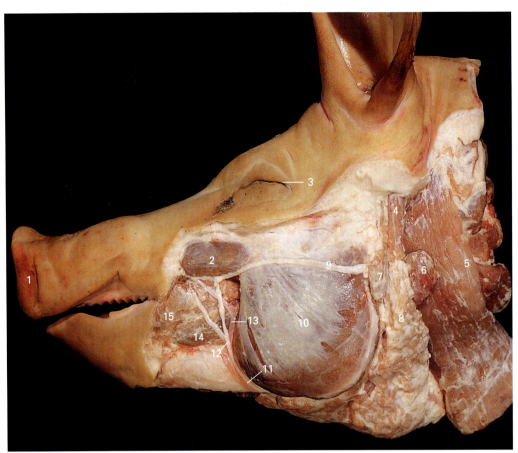

54. Superficial dissection of head of pig, lateral view. Cutaneous muscles have been removed.

1 Rostrum	9 Dorsal buccal branch of facial nerve
2 M. depressor labii superioris	10 M. masseter
3 Orbital fissure	11 Parotid duct
4 M. parotidoauricularis	12 Ventral buccal branch of facial nerve
5 M. brachiocephalicus	13 Facial vein
6 Lateral retropharyngeal lymph node	14 M. depressor labii inferioris
7 Parotid lymph node	15 M. orbicularis oris
8 Parotid gland	

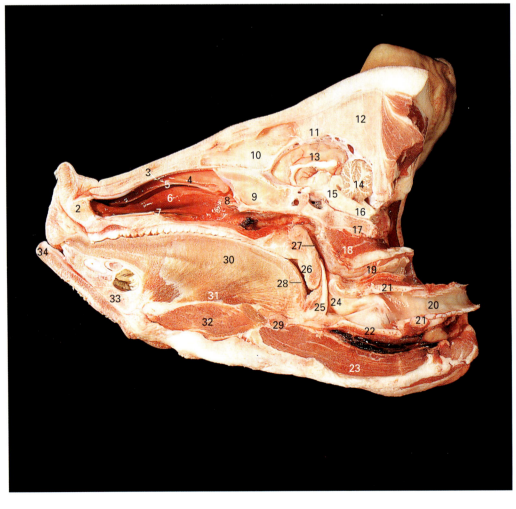

55. Paramedian section through head of pig. Nasal septum has been removed.

1 M. orbicularis oris	18 M. longus capitis
2 Rostral bone	19 Oesophagus
3 Dorsal nasal meatus	20 Trachea
4 Dorsal nasal concha	21 Cricoid cartilage
5 Middle nasal meatus	22 Thyroid cartilage
6 Ventral nasal concha	23 M. sternohyoideus
7 Ventral nasal meatus	24 Arytenoid cartilage
8 Ethmoidal conchae	25 Epiglottis
9 Caudal part of nasal septum	26 Soft palate
10 Frontal sinus	27 Nasopharynx
11 Frontal bone	28 Oropharynx
12 Parietal bone	29 Basihyoid bone
13 Cerebral hemisphere	30 Tongue
14 Cerebellum	31 M. genioglossus
15 Mesencephalon	32 M. geniohyoideus
16 Medulla oblongata	33 Mandible
17 Occipital bone	34 Lower lip

3 Spinal Column

The osteology of the vertebral column is illustrated using bone specimens and the associated musculature is shown on dissected specimens.

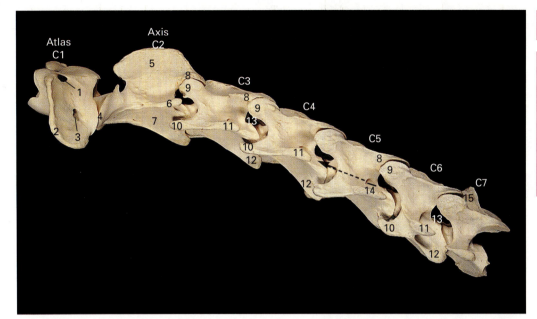

56. Cervical vertebrae (C1–C7) of horse, lateral view.

Atlas (C1)
1 Alar foramen
2 Transverse process (wing)
3 Transverse foramen

Axis (C2)
4 Cranial articular process
5 Spinous process
6 Transverse process
7 Body

C3–C7
8 Caudal articular process
9 Cranial articular process
10 Ventral tubercle of transverse process
11 Dorsal tubercle of transverse process
12 Ventral crest
13 Intervertebral foramen
14 Transverse foramen
15 Spinous process

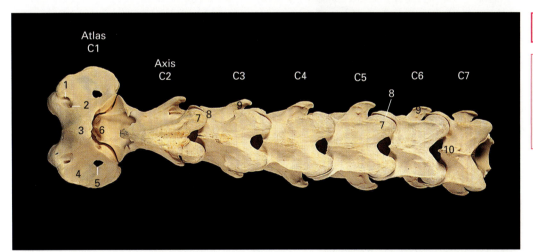

57. Cervical vertebrae (C1–C7) of horse, dorsal view.

Atlas (C1)
1 Alar foramen
2 Lateral vertebral foramen
3 Dorsal arch
4 Transverse process (wing)
5 Transverse foramen

C2–C7
6 Dens (odontoid process) of axis
7 Caudal articular process
8 Cranial articular process
9 Transverse process
10 Spinous process

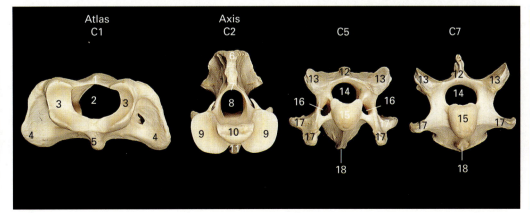

58. Atlas (C1), axis (C2), fifth (C5) and seventh (C7) cervical vertebrae of horse, cranial view.

Atlas (C1)
1 Dorsal arch
2 Vertebral foramen
3 Cranial articular cavity
4 Transverse process (wing)
5 Ventral tubercle

Axis (C2)
6 Spinous process
7 Arch
8 Vertebral foramen

9 Cranial articular process
10 Dens
11 Ventral crest

C5, C7
12 Spinous process
13 Cranial articular process
14 Vertebral foramen
15 Body
16 Transverse foramen
17 Transverse process
18 Ventral crest

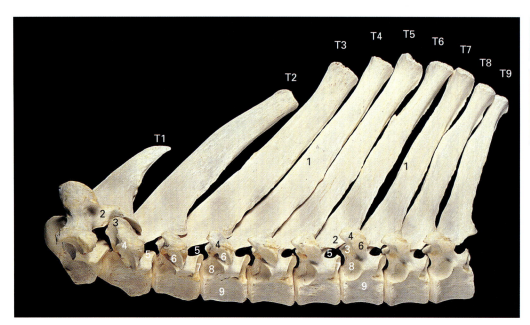

1 Spinous process
2 Caudal articular process
3 Cranial articular process
4 Transverse process
5 Intervertebral foramen
6 Facet for tubercle of rib
7 Caudal costal fovea
8 Cranial costal fovea
9 Body

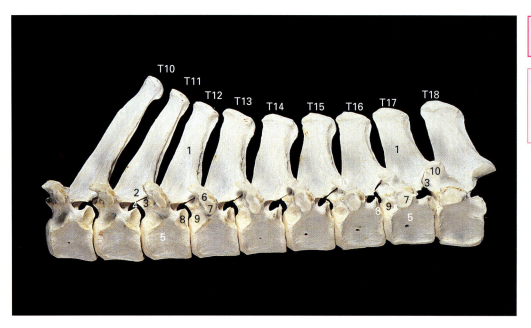

60. Tenth to eighteenth thoracic vertebrae (T10–T18) of horse, lateral view.

1 Spinous process
2 Caudal articular process
3 Cranial articular process
4 Intervertebral foramen
5 Body
6 Transverse process
7 Facet for tubercle of rib
8 Caudal costal fovea
9 Cranial costal fovea
10 Mamillary process

61. First (T1), fifth (T5), twelfth (T12) and eighteenth (T18) thoracic vertebrae of horse, cranial view.

1 Spinous process
2 Cranial articular process
3 Vertebral foramen
4 Transverse process
5 Body
6 Caudal costal fovea
7 Facet for tubercle of rib
8 Mamillary process
9 Ventral tubercle

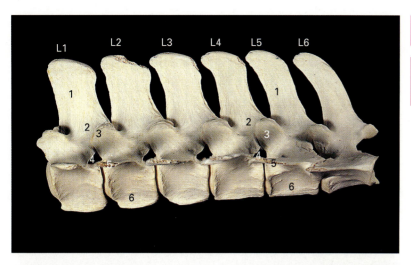

62. Lumbar vertebrae (L1–L6) of horse, lateral view.

1 Spinous process	4 Intervertebral foramen
2 Caudal articular process	5 Transverse process
3 Cranial articular process	6 Body

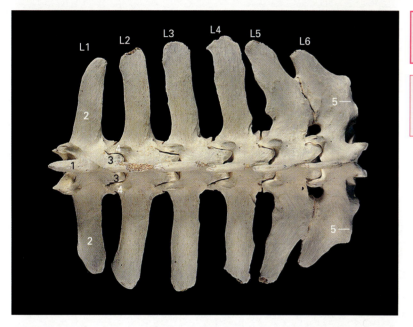

63. Lumbar vertebrae (L1–L6) of horse, dorsal view. Note fusion of transverse processes of fifth and sixth lumbar vertebrae.

1 Spinous process	5 Surface of transverse
2 Transverse process	process for articulation
3 Caudal articular process	with wing of sacrum
4 Cranial articular process	

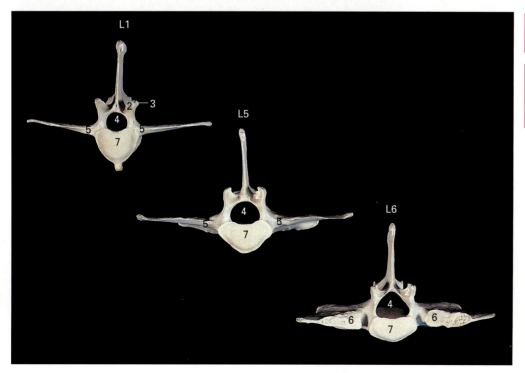

64. First (L1), fifth (L5) and sixth (L6) lumbar vertebrae of horse, cranial view.

1 Spinous process	5 Transverse process
2 Cranial articular process	6 Articular surface of
3 Mamillary process	transverse process
4 Vertebral foramen	7 Body

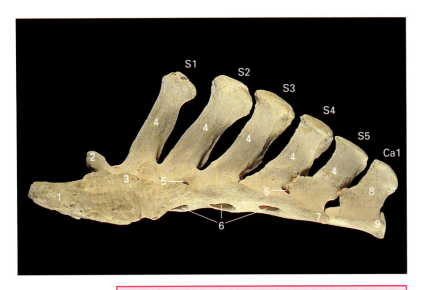

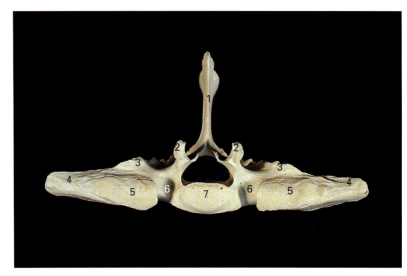

65. Sacrum (S1–S5) and first caudal (Ca1) vertebra of horse, lateral view.

1 Auricular surface	7 Transverse process of sacrum
2 Articular process	
3 Wing	8 Spinous process of first caudal vertebra
4 Spinous process of sacral vertebra	
5 Dorsal sacral foramen	9 Transverse process of first caudal vertebra
6 Ventral sacral foramen	

66. Sacrum of horse, cranial view.

1 Spinous process	5 Articular surface of wing
2 Articular process	6 Notch
3 Lateral crest	7 Body
4 Wing	

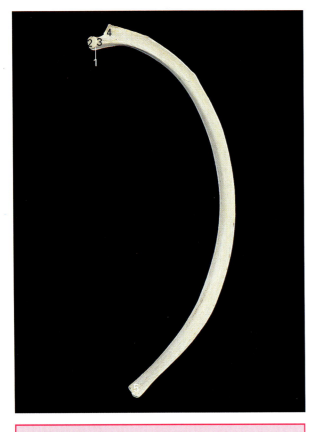

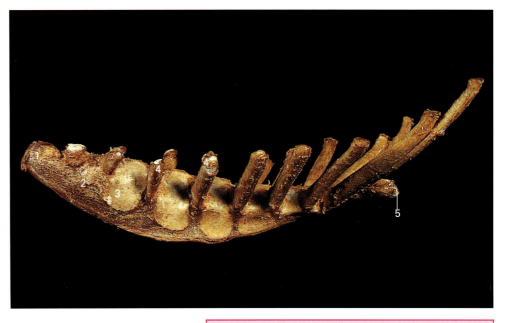

68. Sternum of horse, lateral view.

1 Cartilage of manubrium	4 Costal cartilage
2 Manubrium	5 Xiphoid cartilage
3 Second sternebra	

67. Left eighth rib of horse, cranial view.

1 Costal groove	4 Tubercle
2 Head	5 Sternal extremity
3 Neck	

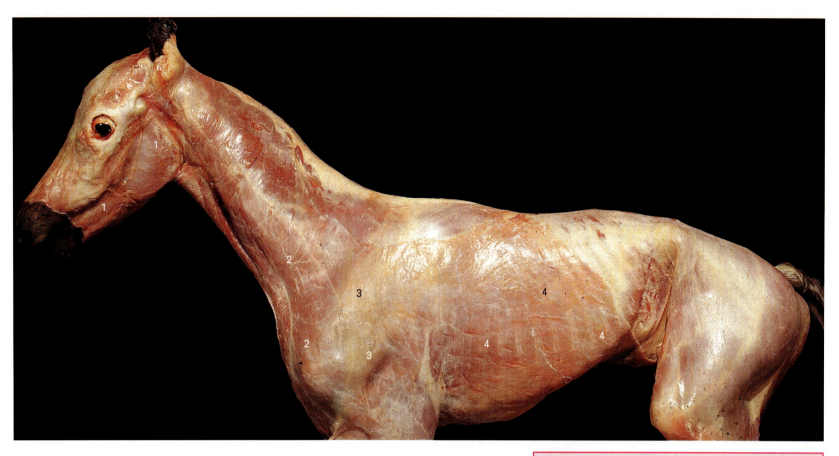

69. Cutaneous musculature of foal, lateral view.

1 M. cutaneus fasciei, part of M. platysma	3 M. cutaneus omobrachialis
2 M. cutaneus colli, part of M. platysma	4 M. cutaneus trunci

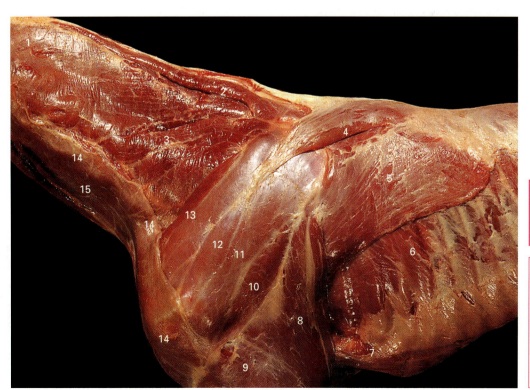

70. Superficial dissection of musculature of neck, shoulder and thoracic wall of foal, lateral view. The cutaneous muscles and cervical part of the M. trapezius have been removed.

1 M. splenius	9 M. triceps brachii, lateral head
2 M. rhomboideus cervicis	10 M. deltoideus
3 M. serratus ventralis cervicis	11 M. infraspinatus
4 M. trapezius, thoracic part	12 M. supraspinatus
5 M. latissimus dorsi	13 M. subclavius
6 M. intercostales externi	14 M. brachiocephalicus
7 M. pectoralis ascendens	15 M. sternocephalicus
8 M. triceps brachii, long head	

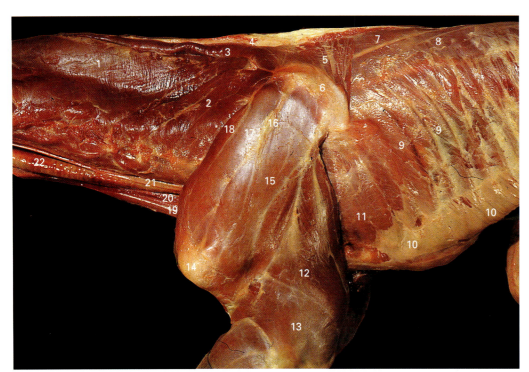

1 M. splenius
2 M. serratus ventralis cervicis
3 M. rhomboideus cervicis
4 Nuchal ligament
5 M. rhomboideus thoracis
6 Scapular cartilage
7 M. spinalis thoracis
8 M. longissimus thoracis
9 M. intercostales externi
10 M. obliquus externus abdominis
11 M. serratus ventralis thoracis
12 M. triceps brachii, long head
13 M. triceps brachii, lateral head
14 Greater tubercle of humerus
15 M. infraspinatus
16 Spine of scapula
17 M. supraspinatus
18 M. subclavius
19 M. sternohyoideus
20 M. sternothyroideus
21 Oesophagus
22 Trachea

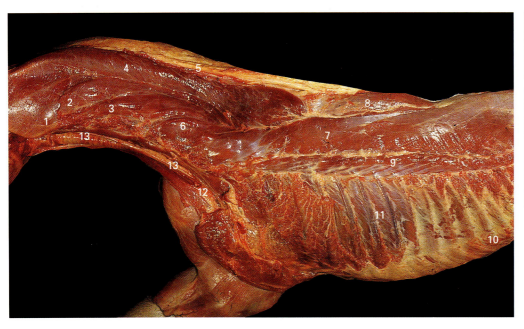

1 M. obliquus capitis caudalis
2 Cut edge of M. longissimus capitis
3 M. longissimus atlantis
4 M. semispinalis capitis
5 Nuchal ligament, funicular part
6 M. longissimus cervicis
7 M. longissimus thoracis
8 M. spinalis thoracis
9 M. iliocostalis thoracis
10 M. obliquus externus abdominis
11 M. intercostales externi
12 M. sternohyoideus and M. sternothyroideus
13 Trachea

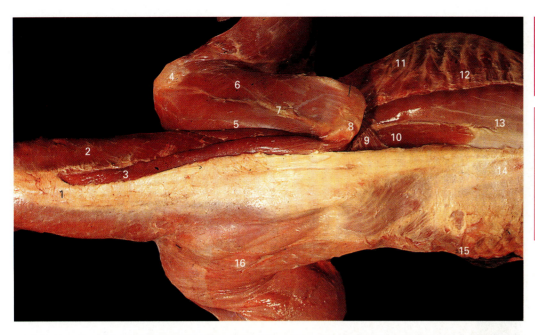

73. Superficial (left side) and deep (right side) dissections of musculature of neck and trunk of foal, dorsal view. The cutaneous muscles, M. trapezius and M. latissimus dorsi have been removed on the right side.

1 Funicular part of nuchal ligament
2 M. splenius
3 M. rhomboideus cervicis
4 Greater tubercle of humerus
5 M. supraspinatus
6 M. infraspinatus
7 Spine of scapula
8 Cartilage of scapula
9 M. rhomboideus thoracis
10 M. spinalis thoracis
11 M. intercostales externi
12 M. serratus dorsalis caudalis
13 M. longissimus thoracis
14 Lumbodorsal fascia
15 M. cutaneus trunci
16 M. cutaneus omobrachialis

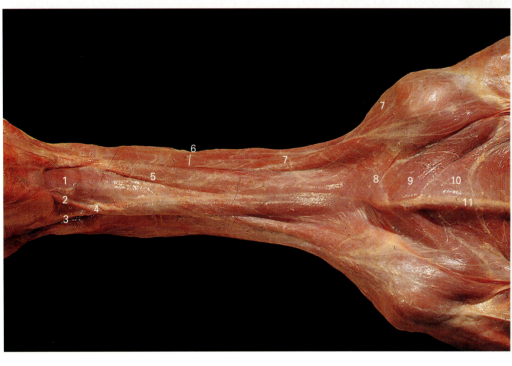

74. Superficial dissection of musculature of neck and pectoral region of foal, ventral view.

1 M. sternohyoideus and M. omohyoideus
2 Maxillary vein
3 Linguofacial vein
4 External jugular vein
5 M. sternocephalicus
6 Jugular groove
7 M. brachiocephalicus
8 M. cutaneus colli
9 M. pectoralis transversus
10 M. pectoralis descendens
11 Sternum

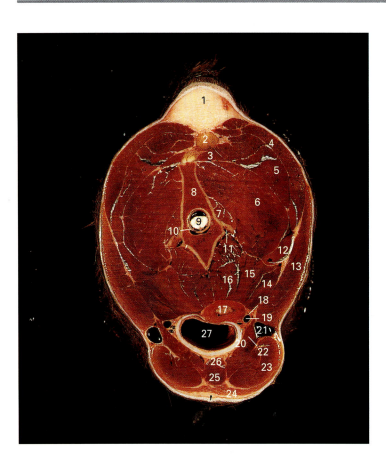

75. Transverse section through neck of horse at the level of the second cervical vertebra, cranial view. The vertebra is slightly twisted.

1 Nuchal adipose body (crest)	12 M. longissimus capitis
2 Nuchal ligament, funicular part	13 M. brachiocephalicus
3 M. rectus capitis dorsalis major	14 M. longissimus atlantis
4 M. splenius	15 M. longus capitis
5 M. semispinalis capitis	16 M. longus colli
6 M. obliquus capitis dorsalis	17 Oesophagus
7 M. multifidus cervicis	18 Vagosympathetic trunk
8 Second cervical vertebra (axis)	19 Common carotid artery
9 Spinal cord	20 Recurrent laryngeal nerve
10 Internal vertebral plexus	21 External jugular vein
11 Vertebral artery and vein	22 M. omohyoideus
	23 M. sternocephalicus
	24 M. cutaneus colli
	25 M. sternohyoideus
	26 M. sternothyroideus
	27 Trachea

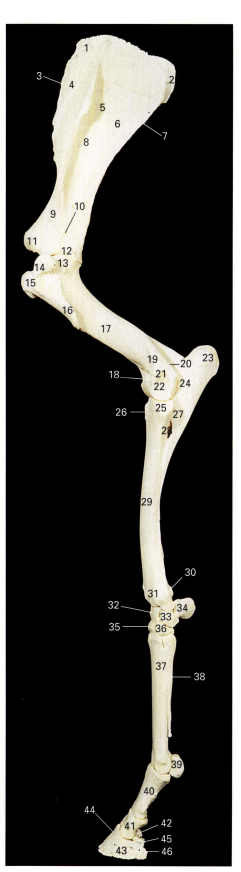

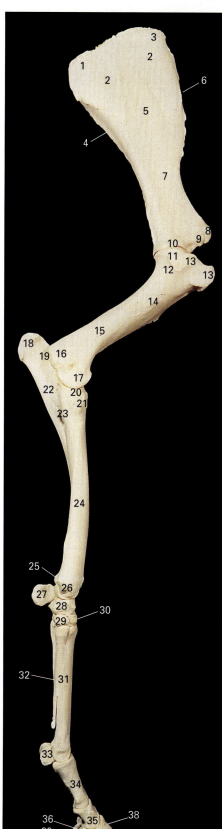

Scapula

1 Cranial angle
2 Caudal angle
3 Cranial border
4 Supraspinous fossa
5 Tuber of scapular spine
6 Infraspinous fossa
7 Caudal border
8 Spine
9 Neck
10 Nutrient foramen
11 Supraglenoid tubercle
12 Glenoid cavity

Humerus

13 Head
14 Greater tubercle
15 Intertuberal groove
16 Deltoid tuberosity
17 Body
18 Radial fossa
19 Lateral supracondyloid crest
20 Olecranon fossa
21 Lateral epicondyle
22 Condyle

Antebrachium

23 Olecranon tuberosity
24 Trochlear notch
25 Capitular fovea
26 Radial tuberosity
27 Body of ulna
28 Interosseous space
29 Body of radius
30 Transverse crest
31 Trochlea

Manus

32 Intermediate carpal bone
33 Ulnar carpal bone
34 Accessory carpal bone
35 Third carpal bone
36 Fourth carpal bone
37 Metacarpal III (cannon bone)
38 Metacarpal IV (lateral splint bone)
39 Proximal sesamoid bone
40 Proximal phalanx
41 Middle phalanx
42 Distal sesamoid (navicular) bone
43 Distal phalanx
44 Extensor process
45 Lateral parietal sulcus
46 Lateral process

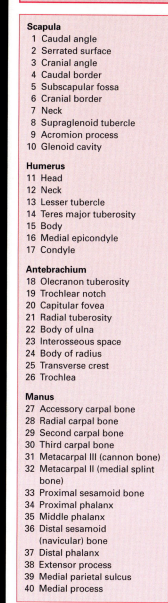

Scapula

1 Caudal angle
2 Serrated surface
3 Cranial angle
4 Caudal border
5 Subscapular fossa
6 Cranial border
7 Neck
8 Supraglenoid tubercle
9 Acromion process
10 Glenoid cavity

Humerus

11 Head
12 Neck
13 Lesser tubercle
14 Teres major tuberosity
15 Body
16 Medial epicondyle
17 Condyle

Antebrachium

18 Olecranon tuberosity
19 Trochlear notch
20 Capitular fovea
21 Radial tuberosity
22 Body of ulna
23 Interosseous space
24 Body of radius
25 Transverse crest
26 Trochlea

Manus

27 Accessory carpal bone
28 Radial carpal bone
29 Second carpal bone
30 Third carpal bone
31 Metacarpal III (cannon bone)
32 Metacarpal II (medial splint bone)
33 Proximal sesamoid bone
34 Proximal phalanx
35 Middle phalanx
36 Distal sesamoid (navicular) bone
37 Distal phalanx
38 Extensor process
39 Medial parietal sulcus
40 Medial process

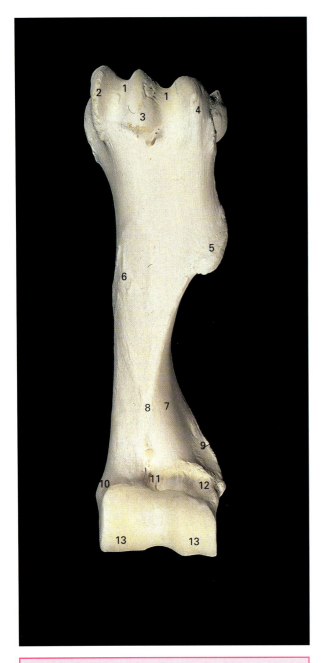

78. Left humerus of horse, cranial view.

1 Intertuberal groove	8 Humeral crest
2 Lesser tubercle	9 Lateral epicondyloid crest
3 Intermediate tubercle	10 Medial epicondyle
4 Greater tubercle	11 Radial fossa
5 Deltoid tuberosity	12 Lateral epicondyle
6 Teres major tuberosity	13 Trochlea
7 M. brachialis (musculospiral) groove	

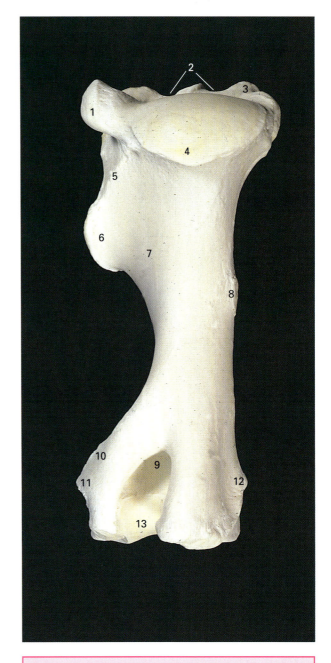

79. Left humerus of horse, caudal view.

1 Greater tubercle	8 Teres major tuberosity
2 Intertuberal groove	9 Olecranon fossa
3 Lesser tubercle	10 Lateral epicondyloid crest
4 Head	11 Lateral epicondyle
5 Tricipital line	12 Medial epicondyle
6 Deltoid tuberosity	13 Trochlea
7 M. brachialis (musculospiral) groove	

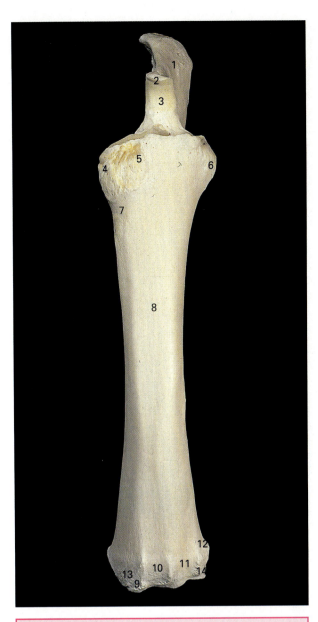

80. Left radius and ulna of horse, cranial view.

Ulna
1 Olecranon tuberosity
2 Anconeal process
3 Trochlear notch

Radius
4 Medial tuberosity
5 Radial tuberosity
6 Lateral tuberosity
7 Groove for M. brachialis
8 Body

9 Groove for tendon of M. abductor digiti I longus
10 Groove for tendon of M. extensor carpi radialis
11 Groove for tendon of M. extensor digitorum communis
12 Groove for tendon of M. extensor digitorum lateralis
13 Medial styloid process
14 Lateral styloid process

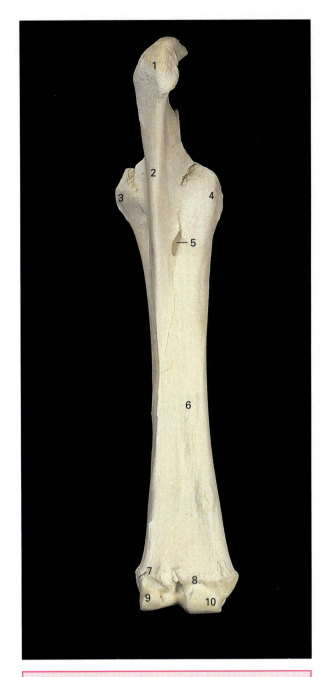

81. Left radius and ulna of horse, caudal view.

Ulna
1 Olecranon tuberosity
2 Body

Radius
3 Lateral tuberosity
4 Medial tuberosity
5 Interosseous space

6 Body
7 Groove for tendon of M. extensor digitorum lateralis
8 Transverse crest
9 Lateral styloid process
10 Medial styloid process

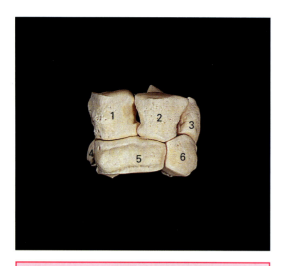

82. Left carpal bones of horse, dorsal view.

1 Radial carpal bone	4 Second carpal bone
2 Intermediate carpal bone	5 Third carpal bone
3 Ulnar carpal bone	6 Fourth carpal bone

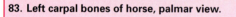

83. Left carpal bones of horse, palmar view.

1 Accessory carpal bone	5 Fourth carpal bone
2 Ulnar carpal bone	6 Third carpal bone
3 Intermediate carpal bone	7 Second carpal bone
4 Radial carpal bone	8 First carpal bone (inconstant)

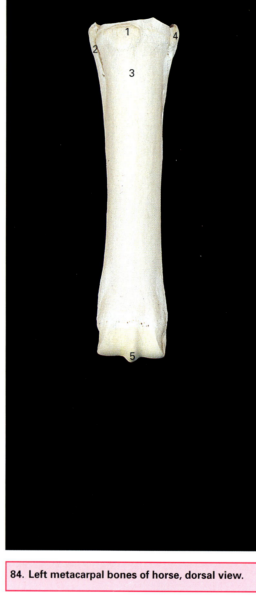

84. Left metacarpal bones of horse, dorsal view.

1 Metacarpal tuberosity	4 Metacarpal IV (lateral splint bone)
2 Metacarpal II (medial splint bone)	5 Sagittal ridge
3 Metacarpal III (cannon bone)	

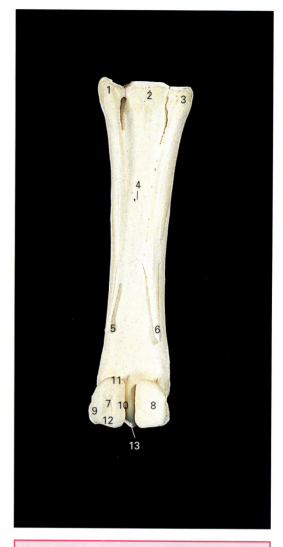

85. Left metacarpal and proximal sesamoid bones of horse, palmar view.

1 Metacarpal IV (lateral splint bone)	7 Lateral proximal sesamoid bone
2 Metacarpal III (cannon bone)	8 Medial proximal sesamoid bone
3 Metacarpal II (medial splint bone)	9 Abaxial surface
4 Nutrient foramen	10 Axial surface
5 Metacarpal IV, distal extremity (button)	11 Apex
6 Metacarpal II, distal extremity (button)	12 Base
	13 Sagittal ridge

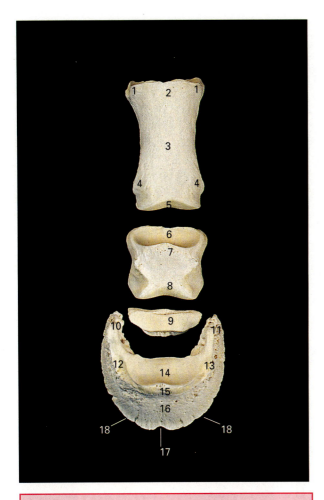

86. Bones of left digit of horse, dorsal view.

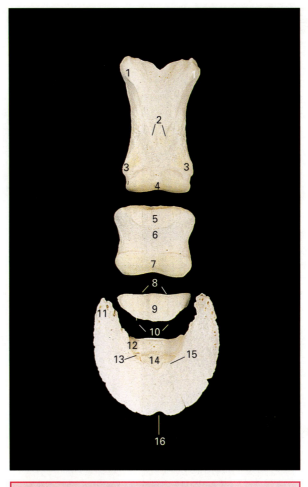

87. Bones of left digit of horse, palmar view.

Proximal phalanx
1 Eminences for attachment of collateral ligaments of metacarpophalangeal joint
2 Eminence for attachment of digital extensor tendons
3 Body
4 Eminences for attachment of collateral ligaments of proximal interphalangeal joint
5 Distal articular surface

Middle phalanx
6 Proximal articular surface
7 Extensor process
8 Distal articular surface

Distal sesamoid (navicular) bone
9 Articular surface

Distal phalanx
10 Medial palmar process
11 Lateral palmar process
12 Medial parietal sulcus
13 Lateral parietal sulcus
14 Articular surface
15 Extensor process
16 Parietal surface
17 Crena
18 Solar border

Proximal phalanx
1 Eminences for attachment of collateral ligaments of metacarpophalangeal joint
2 Triangular rough area
3 Eminences for attachment of collateral ligaments of proximal interphalangeal joint
4 Condyle

Middle phalanx
5 Articular fovea
6 Flexor tuberosity
7 Condyle

Distal sesamoid (navicular) bone
8 Proximal border
9 Flexor surface
10 Distal border

Distal phalanx
11 Lateral palmar process
12 Lateral solar groove
13 Lateral solar foramen
14 Flexor surface
15 Semilunar line
16 Crena

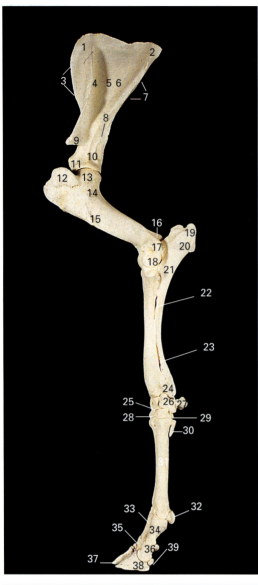
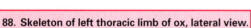
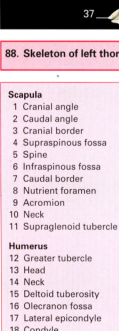

88. Skeleton of left thoracic limb of ox, lateral view.

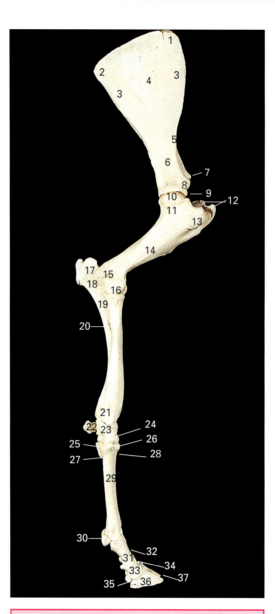

89. Skeleton of left thoracic limb of ox, medial view.

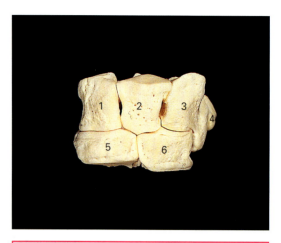

90. Left carpal bones of ox, dorsal view.

1 Radial carpal bone
2 Intermediate carpal bone
3 Ulnar carpal bone
4 Accessory carpal bone
5 Second and third carpal bones (fused)
6 Fourth carpal bone

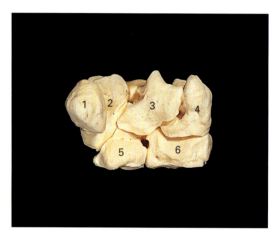

91. Left carpal bones of ox, palmar view.

1 Accessory carpal bone
2 Ulnar carpal bone
3 Intermediate carpal bone
4 Radial carpal bone
5 Fourth carpal bone
6 Second and third carpal bones (fused)

Scapula
1 Cranial angle
2 Caudal angle
3 Cranial border
4 Supraspinous fossa
5 Spine
6 Infraspinous fossa
7 Caudal border
8 Nutrient foramen
9 Acromion
10 Neck
11 Supraglenoid tubercle

Humerus
12 Greater tubercle
13 Head
14 Neck
15 Deltoid tuberosity
16 Olecranon fossa
17 Lateral epicondyle
18 Condyle

Antebrachium
19 Olecranon tuberosity
20 Olecranon
21 Body of ulna
22 Proximal interosseous space of forearm
23 Distal interosseous space of forearm
24 Styloid process

Manus
25 Intermediate carpal bone
26 Ulnar carpal bone
27 Accessory carpal bone
28 Second and third carpal bones (fused)
29 Fourth carpal bone
30 Metacarpal V
31 Metacarpals III and IV (fused)
32 Proximal sesamoid bone
33 Proximal phalanx, digit III
34 Proximal phalanx, digit IV
35 Middle phalanx, digit III
36 Middle phalanx, digit IV
37 Distal phalanx, digit III
38 Distal phalanx, digit IV
39 Distal sesamoid bone, digit IV

Scapula
1 Cranial angle
2 Caudal angle
3 Facies serrata
4 Fossa subscapularis
5 Scapular notch
6 Neck
7 Acromion
8 Supraglenoid tubercle
9 Coracoid process

Humerus
10 Head
11 Neck
12 Greater tubercle
13 Lesser tubercle
14 Teres major tuberosity
15 Medial epicondyle
16 Condyle

Antebrachium
17 Olecranon tuber
18 Olecranon
19 Body of ulna
20 Proximal interosseous space of forearm
21 Styloid process

Manus
22 Accessory carpal bone
23 Radial carpal bone
24 Intermediate carpal bone
25 Fourth carpal bone
26 Second and third carpal bones (fused)
27 Metacarpal V
28 Metacarpal tuberosity
29 Metacarpals III and IV (fused)
30 Proximal sesamoid bone
31 Proximal phalanx, digit III
32 Proximal phalanx, digit IV
33 Middle phalanx, digit III
34 Middle phalanx, digit IV
35 Distal sesamoid bone, digit III
36 Distal phalanx, digit III
37 Distal phalanx, digit IV

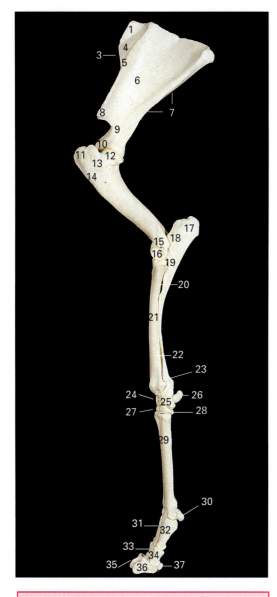

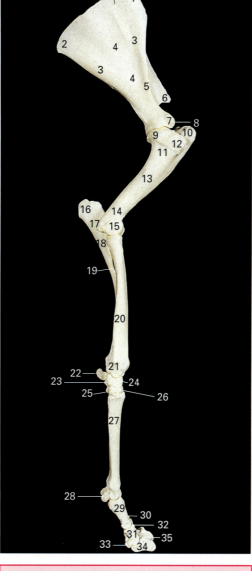

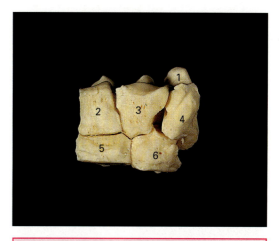

94. Left carpal bones of sheep, dorsal view.

1 Accessory carpal bone	4 Ulnar carpal bone
2 Radial carpal bone	5 Second and third
3 Intermediate carpal	carpal bones (fused)
bone	6 Fourth carpal bone

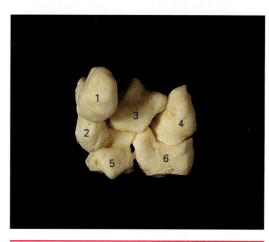

95. Left carpal bones of sheep, palmar view.

1 Accessory carpal bone	4 Radial carpal bone
2 Ulnar carpal bone	5 Fourth carpal bone
3 Intermediate carpal	6 Second and third
bone	carpal bones (fused)

92. Skeleton of left thoracic limb of sheep, lateral view.

Scapula
1 Cranial angle
2 Caudal angle
3 Cranial border
4 Supraspinous fossa
5 Spine
6 Infraspinous fossa
7 Caudal border
8 Acromion
9 Neck
10 Supraglenoid tubercle

Humerus
11 Greater tubercle
12 Head
13 Neck
14 Deltoid tuberosity
15 Lateral epicondyle
16 Condyle

Antebrachium
17 Olecranon tuberosity
18 Olecranon
19 Body of ulna
20 Proximal interosseous space of forearm
21 Body of radius
22 Distal interosseous space of forearm
23 Styloid process

Manus
24 Intermediate carpal bone
25 Ulnar carpal bone
26 Accessory carpal bone
27 Second and third carpal bones (fused)
28 Fourth carpal bone
29 Metacarpals III and IV (fused)
30 Proximal sesamoid bone
31 Proximal phalanx, digit III
32 Proximal phalanx, digit IV
33 Middle phalanx, digit III
34 Middle phalanx, digit IV
35 Distal phalanx, digit III
36 Distal phalanx, digit IV
37 Distal sesamoid bone, digit IV

93. Skeleton of left thoracic limb of sheep, medial view.

Scapula
1 Cranial angle
2 Caudal angle
3 Facies serrata
4 Subscapular fossa
5 Scapular notch
6 Acromion
7 Supraglenoid tubercle
8 Coracoid process

Humerus
9 Head
10 Greater tubercle
11 Neck
12 Lesser tubercle
13 Teres major tuberosity
14 Medial epicondyle
15 Condyle

Antebrachium
16 Olecranon tuberosity
17 Olecranon
18 Body of ulna
19 Proximal interosseous space of forearm
20 Body of radius
21 Styloid process

Manus
22 Accessory carpal bone
23 Ulnar carpal bone
24 Intermediate carpal bone
25 Fourth carpal bone
26 Second and third carpal bones (fused)
27 Metacarpals III and IV (fused)
28 Proximal sesamoid bone
29 Proximal phalanx, digit III
30 Proximal phalanx, digit IV
31 Middle phalanx, digit III
32 Middle phalanx, digit IV
33 Distal sesamoid bone, digit III
34 Distal phalanx, digit III
35 Distal phalanx, digit IV

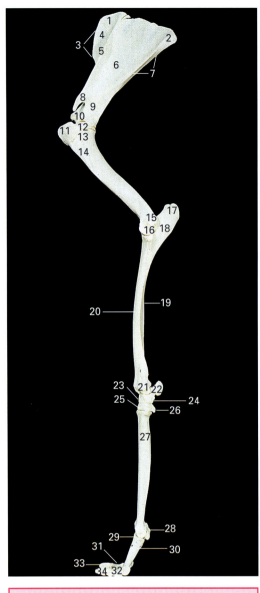

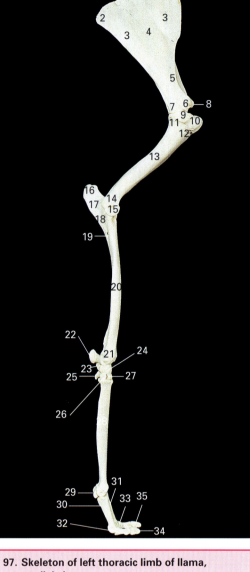

97. Skeleton of left thoracic limb of llama, medial view.

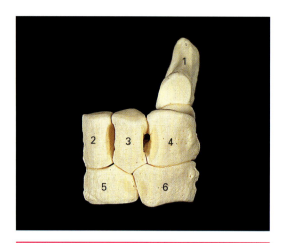

98. Left carpal bones of llama, dorsal view.

1	Accessory carpal bone	4	Ulnar carpal bone
2	Radial carpal bone	5	Third carpal bone
3	Intermediate carpal bone	6	Fourth carpal bone

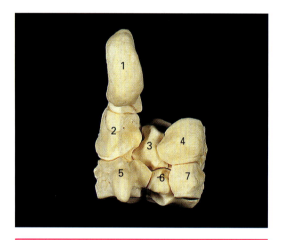

99. Left carpal bones of llama, palmar view.

1	Accessory carpal bone	4	Radial carpal bone
2	Ulnar carpal bone	5	Fourth carpal bone
3	Intermediate carpal bone	6	Third carpal bone
		7	Second carpal bone

Scapula
1 Cranial angle
2 Caudal angle
3 Cranial border
4 Supraspinous fossa
5 Spine
6 Infraspinous fossa
7 Caudal border
8 Acromion
9 Neck
10 Supraglenoid tubercle

Humerus
11 Greater tubercle
12 Head
13 Neck
14 Deltoid tuberosity
15 Lateral epicondyle
16 Condyle

Antebrachium
17 Olecranon tuberosity
18 Olecranon
19 Body of ulna
20 Body of radius
21 Styloid process

Manus
22 Accessory carpal bone
23 Intermediate carpal bone
24 Ulnar carpal bone
25 Third carpal bone
26 Fourth carpal bone
27 Metacarpals III and IV (fused)
28 Proximal sesamoid bone
29 Proximal phalanx, digit III
30 Proximal phalanx, digit IV
31 Middle phalanx, digit III
32 Middle phalanx, digit IV
33 Distal phalanx, digit III
34 Distal phalanx, digit IV

Scapula
1 Cranial angle
2 Caudal angle
3 Facies serrata
4 Subscapular fossa
5 Scapular notch
6 Acromion
7 Supraglenoid tubercle
8 Coracoid process

Humerus
9 Head
10 Greater tubercle
11 Neck
12 Lesser tubercle
13 Body
14 Medial epicondyle
15 Condyle

Antebrachium
16 Olecranon tuberosity
17 Olecranon
18 Body of ulna
19 Proximal interosseous space of forearm
20 Body of radius
21 Styloid process

Manus
22 Accessory carpal bone
23 Ulnar carpal bone
24 Radial carpal bone
25 Fourth carpal bone
26 Second carpal bone
27 Third carpal bone
28 Metacarpals III and IV (fused)
29 Proximal sesamoid bone
30 Proximal phalanx, digit III
31 Proximal phalanx, digit IV
32 Middle phalanx, digit III
33 Middle phalanx, digit IV
34 Distal phalanx, digit III
35 Distal phalanx, digit IV

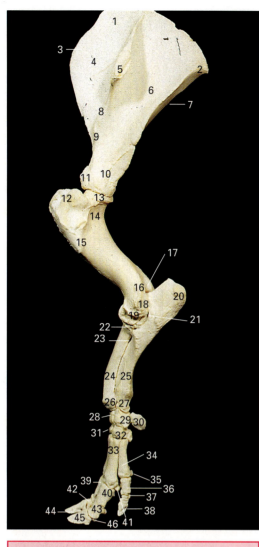

Scapula
1 Cranial angle
2 Caudal angle
3 Cranial border
4 Supraspinous fossa
5 Tuber of scapular spine
6 Infraspinous fossa
7 Caudal border
8 Spine
9 Acromion
10 Neck
11 Supraglenoid tubercle

Humerus
12 Greater tubercle
13 Head
14 Neck
15 Deltoid tuberosity
16 Lateral supracondyloid crest
17 Olecranon fossa
18 Lateral epicondyle
19 Condyle

Antebrachium
20 Olecranon tuberosity
21 Trochlear notch
22 Capitular fovea
23 Interosseous space
24 Body of radius
25 Body of ulna
26 Trochlea
27 Styloid process

Manus
28 Intermediate carpal bone
29 Ulnar carpal bone
30 Accessory carpal bone
31 Third carpal bone
32 Fourth carpal bone
33 Metacarpal IV
34 Metacarpal V
35 Proximal sesamoid bone, digit V
36 Proximal phalanx, digit V
37 Middle phalanx, digit V
38 Distal phalanx, digit V
39 Proximal phalanx, digit III
40 Proximal phalanx, digit IV
41 Proximal sesamoid bone, digit IV
42 Middle phalanx, digit III
43 Middle phalanx, digit IV
44 Distal phalanx, digit III
45 Distal phalanx, digit IV
46 Distal sesamoid bone, digit IV

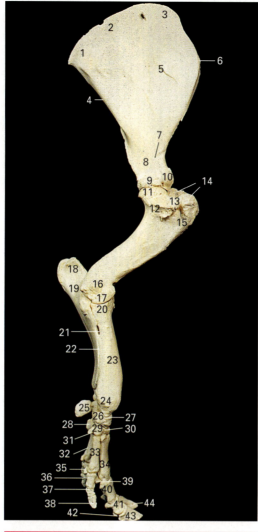

Scapula
1 Caudal angle
2 Serrated surface
3 Cranial angle
4 Caudal border
5 Subscapular fossa
6 Cranial border
7 Vascular groove
8 Neck
9 Glenoid cavity
10 Supraglenoid tubercle

Humerus
11 Head
12 Neck
13 Lesser tubercle
14 Greater tubercle
15 Intertuberal groove
16 Medial epicondyle
17 Condyle

Antebrachium
18 Olecranon
19 Trochlear notch
20 Capitular fovea
21 Interosseous space
22 Body of ulna
23 Body of radius
24 Styloid process

Manus
25 Accessory carpal bone
26 Radial carpal bone
27 Intermediate carpal bone
28 Second carpal bone
29 Third carpal bone
30 Fourth carpal bone
31 First carpal bone
32 Metacarpal V
33 Metacarpal II
34 Metacarpal III
35 Proximal sesamoid bone, digit II
36 Proximal phalanx, digit II
37 Middle phalanx, digit II
38 Distal phalanx, digit II
39 Proximal sesamoid bone, digit III
40 Proximal phalanx, digit III
41 Middle phalanx, digit III
42 Distal sesamoid bone, digit III
43 Distal phalanx, digit III
44 Distal phalanx, digit IV

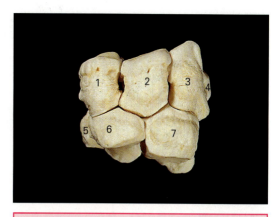

1 Radial carpal bone
2 Intermediate carpal bone
3 Ulnar carpal bone
4 Accessory carpal bone
5 Second carpal bone
6 Third carpal bone
7 Fourth carpal bone

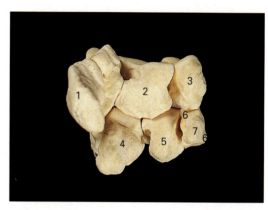

1 Accessory carpal bone
2 Intermediate carpal bone
3 Radial carpal bone
4 Fourth carpal bone
5 Third carpal bone
6 Second carpal bone
7 First carpal bone

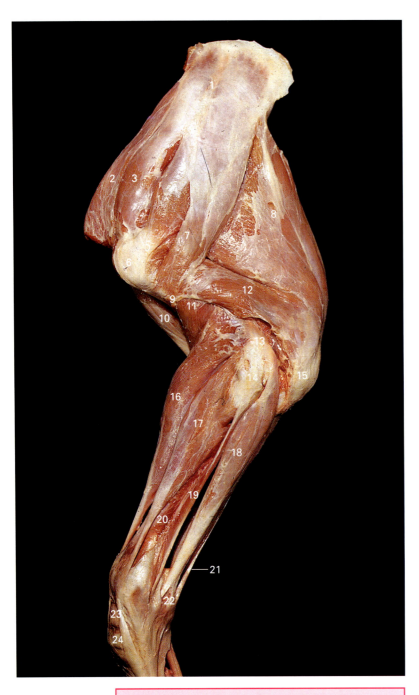

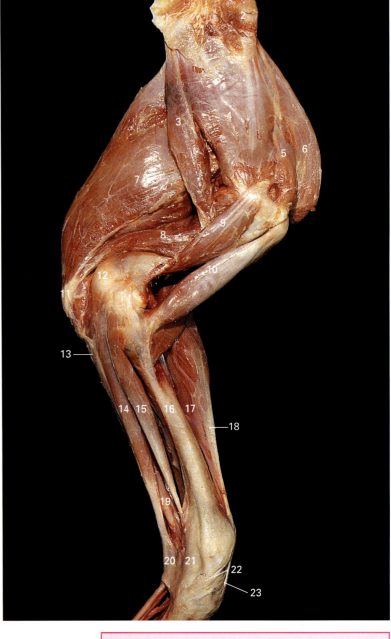

104. Superficial dissection of musculature of left thoracic limb of horse, lateral view.

105. Dissection of musculature of left thoracic limb of horse, medial view. The M. tensor fascia antebrachii has been removed.

1 Spine of scapula	15 Olecranon tuberosity
2 M. subclavius	16 M. extensor carpi radialis
3 M. supraspinatus	17 M. extensor digitorum
4 M. infraspinatus	communis
5 Tendon of M. infraspinatus	18 M. extensor carpi ulnaris
6 Greater tubercle of	(M. ulnaris lateralis)
humerus	19 M. extensor digitorum
7 M. deltoideus	lateralis
8 M. triceps brachii, long	20 M. abductor digiti I
head	longus
9 Deltoid tuberosity	21 M. flexor carpi ulnaris
10 M. biceps brachii	22 Accessory carpal bone
11 M. brachialis	23 Intermediate carpal bone
12 M. triceps brachii, lateral	24 Third carpal bone
head	
13 Lateral epicondyle of	
humerus	
14 Olecranon	

1 Attachment of M.	13 M. flexor digitorum
rhomboideus	profundus, ulnar head
2 Attachment of M. serratus	14 M. flexor carpi ulnaris
ventralis	15 M. flexor carpi radialis
3 M. teres major	16 Radius
4 M. subscapularis	17 M. extensor carpi radialis
5 M. supraspinatus	18 Lacertus fibrosus
6 M. subclavius	19 M. flexor digitorum
7 M. triceps brachii, long	superficialis
head	20 Carpal flexor retinaculum
8 M. triceps brachii, medial	21 Medial collateral carpal
head	ligament
9 M. coracobrachialis	22 Tendon of M. abductor
10 M. biceps brachii	digiti I longus
11 Olecranon tuberosity	23 Tendon of M. extensor
12 Medial epicondyle of	carpi radialis
humerus	

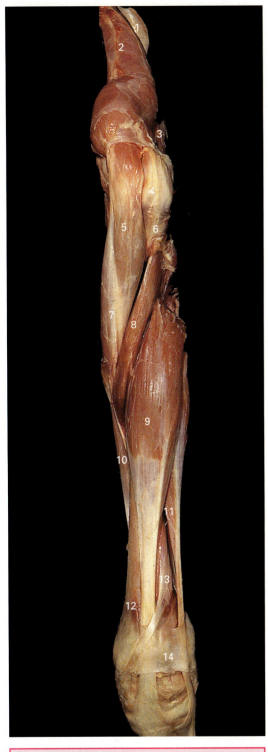

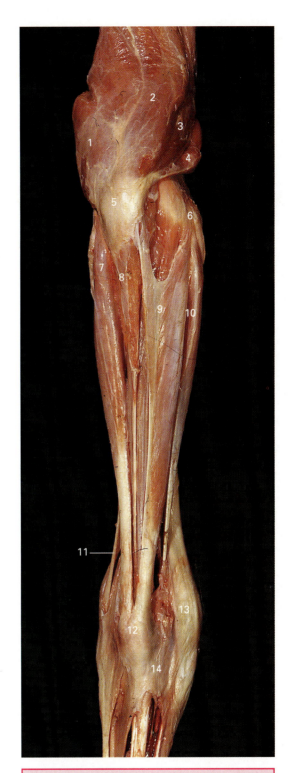

106. Superficial dissection of musculature of left thoracic limb of horse, cranial view. The pectoral muscles and M. subclavius have been removed.

1 Scapular cartilage	9 M. extensor carpi radialis
2 M. supraspinatus	10 M. flexor carpi radialis
3 M. deltoideus	11 M. extensor digitorum communis
4 Greater tubercle of humerus	12 Radius
5 M. biceps brachii	13 M. abductor digiti I longus
6 Deltoid tuberosity	14 Extensor retinaculum of carpus
7 Tendinous intersection of M. biceps brachii	
8 M. brachialis	

107. Superficial dissection of musculature of left thoracic limb of horse, caudal view.

1 M. triceps brachii, lateral head	8 M. flexor digitorum profundus, ulnar head
2 M. triceps brachii, long head	9 M. flexor carpi ulnaris
3 M. triceps brachii, medial head	10 M. flexor carpi radialis
4 M. tensor fascia antebrachii	11 Tendon of M. extensor digitorum lateralis
5 Olecranon tuberosity	12 Accessory carpal bone
6 M. flexor carpi radialis	13 Medial collateral carpal ligament
7 M. extensor carpi ulnaris (M. ulnaris lateralis)	14 Carpal flexor retinaculum

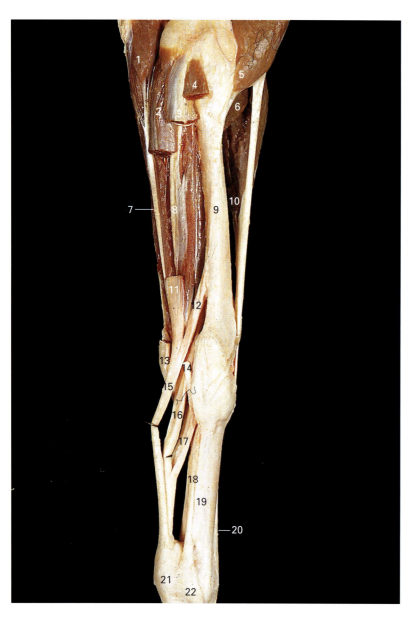

108. Deep dissection of left thoracic limb of horse, medial view. The M. flexor carpi radialis, M. flexor carpi ulnaris and M. flexor digitorum superficialis have been removed. The tendons of the M. flexor digitorum superficialis and M. flexor digitorum profundus have been retracted to expose the accessory ligaments.

1 M. flexor digitorum profundus, ulnar head
2 Stump of M. flexor digitorum superficialis
3 Stump of M. flexor carpi ulnaris
4 Stump of M. flexor carpi radialis
5 M. biceps brachii
6 Lacertus fibrosus
7 Tendon of M. flexor digitorum profundus, ulnar head
8 M. flexor digitorum profundus, humeral head
9 Radius
10 M. extensor carpi radialis
11 Tendon of M. flexor digitorum superficialis
12 Accessory ligament of M. flexor digitorum superficialis (proximal check ligament)
13 Accessory carpal bone
14 Cut edge of tendon of M. flexor carpi radialis
15 Tendon of M. flexor digitorum superficialis
16 Tendon of M. flexor digitorum profundus
17 Accessory ligament of M. flexor digitorum profundus (distal check ligament)
18 M. interosseus medius (suspensory ligament)
19 Metacarpal III (cannon bone)
20 Tendon of M. extensor digitorum communis
21 Superficial transverse metacarpal ligament (palmar annular ligament)
22 Medial extensor branch of M. interosseus medius to tendon of M. extensor digitorum communis

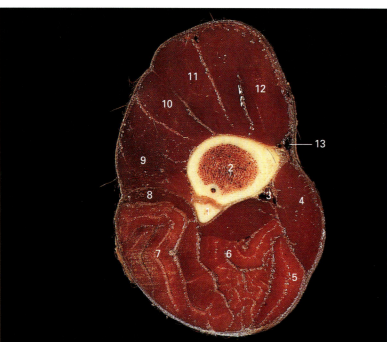

109. Transverse section through left antebrachium of horse, distal view.

1 Ulna
2 Radius
3 Median vessels and nerve
4 M. flexor carpi radialis
5 M. flexor carpi ulnaris
6 M. flexor digitorum superficialis
7 M. flexor digitorum profundus, humeral head
8 M. flexor digitorum profundus, ulnar head
9 M. extensor carpi ulnaris (M. ulnaris lateralis)
10 M. extensor digitorum lateralis
11 M. extensor digitorum communis
12 M. extensor carpi radialis
13 Cephalic vein

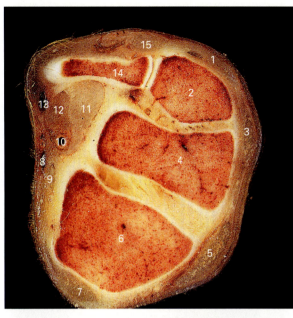

110. Transverse section through left carpus of horse at level of proximal row of carpal bones, distal view.

1 Tendon of M. extensor digitorum lateralis	10 Medial palmar artery and nerve
2 Ulnar carpal bone	11 Tendon of M. flexor digitorum profundus
3 Tendon of M. extensor digitorum communis	12 Tendon of M. flexor digitorum superficialis
4 Intermediate carpal bone	13 Lateral palmar vessels and nerve
5 Tendon of M. extensor carpi radialis	14 Accessory carpal bone
6 Radial carpal bone	15 Tendon of M. extensor carpi ulnaris
7 Tendon of M. abductor digiti I longus	
8 Medial palmar vein	
9 Tendon of M. flexor carpi radialis	

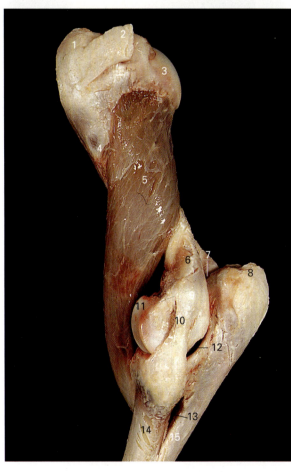

111. Deep dissection of left cubital joint of horse, lateral view.

1 Greater tubercle	9 Lateral epicondyle
2 Tendon of M. infraspinatus	10 Lateral collateral ligament
3 Head of humerus	11 Trochlea
4 Deltoid tuberosity	12 Trochlear notch of ulna
5 M. brachialis	13 Interosseous space
6 Lateral epicondyloid crest	14 Radius
7 Olecranon fossa	15 Ulna
8 Olecranon tuberosity	

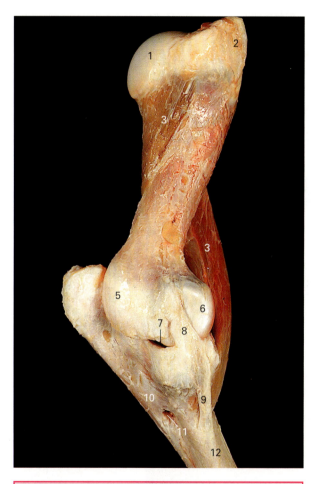

112. Deep dissection of left cubital joint of horse, medial view.

1 Head of humerus	8 Short part of medial collateral ligament
2 Lesser tubercle	9 Long part of medial collateral ligament
3 M. brachialis	
4 Olecranon tuberosity	10 Ulna
5 Medial epicondyle	11 Interosseous space
6 Trochlea	12 Radius
7 Capitular fovea	

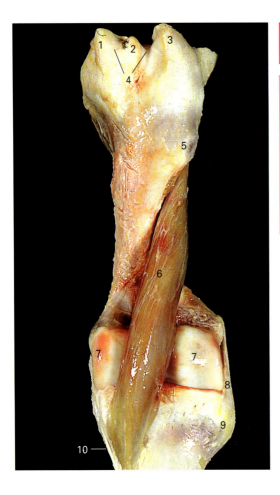

113. Deep dissection of left cubital joint of horse, cranial view.

1 Lesser tubercle	9 Attachment site of
2 Intermediate tubercle	M. extensor
3 Greater tubercle	digitorum
4 Intertuberal groove	communis and
5 Deltoid tuberosity	M. extensor
6 M. brachialis	digitorum lateralis
7 Trochlea	10 Long part of medial
8 Lateral collateral	collateral ligament
ligament	

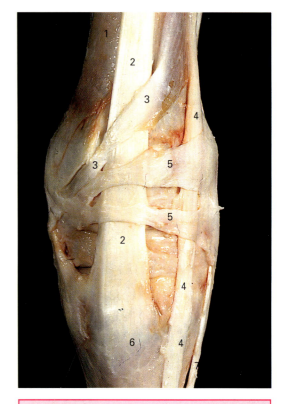

115. Superficial dissection of left carpus of horse, dorsal view.

1 Radius	5 Extensor retinaculum
2 Tendon of M. extensor	6 Metacarpal
carpi radialis	tuberosity
3 Tendon of M. abductor	7 Tendon of
digiti I longus	M. extensor
4 Tendon of M. extensor	digitorum lateralis
digitorum communis	

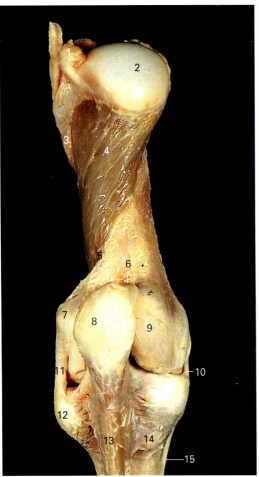

114. Deep dissection of left cubital joint of horse, caudal view.

1 Greater tubercle	11 Lateral collateral
2 Head of humerus	ligament
3 Deltoid tuberosity	12 Attachment site of
4 M. brachialis	M. extensor
5 Lateral epicondyloid	digitorum communis
crest	and M. extensor
6 Olecranon fossa	digitorum lateralis
7 Lateral epicondyle	13 Ulna
8 Olecranon tuberosity	14 Radius
9 Medial epicondyle	15 Long part of medial
10 Short part of medial	collateral ligament
collateral ligament	

Horse

4 Thoracic Limb and Digit

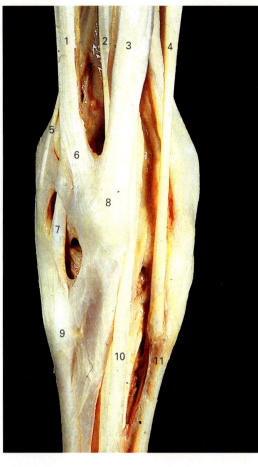

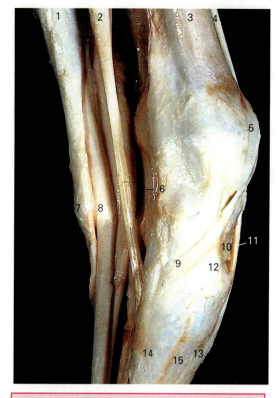

116. Superficial dissection of left carpus of horse, palmar view. Flexor retinaculum has been removed.

1 Tendon of M. extensor carpi ulnaris (M. ulnaris lateralis)
2 Tendon of M. flexor digitorum profundus
3 Tendon of M. flexor carpi ulnaris
4 Tendon of M. flexor carpi radialis
5 Tendon of M. extensor digitorum lateralis
6 Tendon of M. extensor carpi ulnaris to accessory carpal bone
7 Tendon of M. extensor carpi ulnaris to metacarpal IV
8 Accessory carpal bone
9 Metacarpal IV (lateral splint bone)
10 Tendon of M. flexor digitorum superficialis
11 Metacarpal II (medial splint bone)

118. Superficial dissection of left carpus of horse, medial view. Flexor retinaculum has been removed to expose contents of the carpal canal.

1 M. flexor carpi ulnaris
2 M. flexor carpi radialis
3 Radius
4 M. extensor carpi radialis
5 Extensor retinaculum of carpus
6 Cut edge of flexor retinaculum
7 Accessory carpal bone
8 Tendon of M. flexor digitorum superficialis passing through carpal canal
9 Tendon of M. abductor digiti I longus
10 Third carpal bone
11 Tendon of M. extensor carpi radialis
12 Medial collateral carpal ligament
13 Metacarpal tuberosity
14 Metacarpal II (medial splint bone)
15 Metacarpal III (cannon bone)

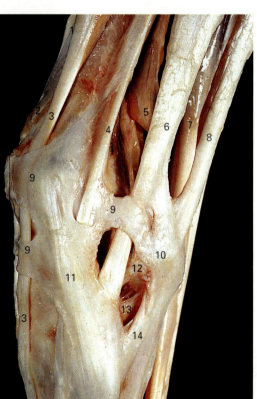

117. Superficial dissection of left carpus of horse, lateral view.

1 Tendon of M. extensor carpi radialis
2 M. abductor digiti I longus
3 Tendon of M. extensor digitorum communis
4 Tendon of M. extensor digitorum lateralis
5 M. flexor digitorum profundus, humeral head
6 Tendon of M. extensor carpi ulnaris (M. ulnaris lateralis)
7 M. flexor digitorum profundus, ulnar head
8 Tendon of M. flexor carpi ulnaris
9 Extensor retinaculum
10 Accessory carpal bone
11 Lateral collateral carpal ligament
12 Accessoriocarpoulnar ligament
13 Accessorioquartal ligament
14 Accessoriometacarpal ligament

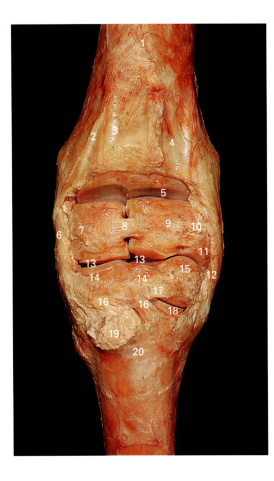

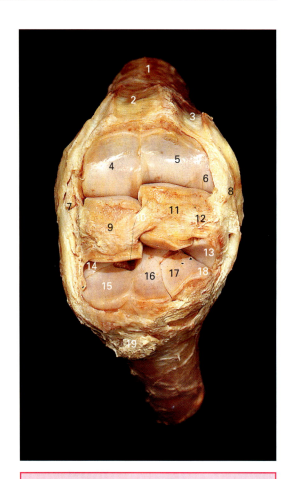

119. Deep dissection of left carpal joint of horse, dorsal view.

1 Radius
2 Groove for tendon of M. abductor digiti I longus
3 Groove for tendon of M. extensor carpi radialis
4 Groove for tendon of M. extensor digitorum communis
5 Antebrachiocarpal joint
6 Medial collateral carpal ligament
7 Radial carpal bone
8 Dorsal intercarpal ligament between radial and intermediate carpal bones
9 Intermediate carpal bone
10 Dorsal intercarpal ligament between intermediate and ulnar carpal bones
11 Ulnar carpal bone
12 Lateral collateral carpal ligament
13 Intercarpal joint
14 Third carpal bone
15 Fourth carpal bone
16 Dorsal carpometacarpal ligament
17 Dorsal intercarpal ligament between third and fourth carpal bones
18 Carpometacarpal joint
19 Metacarpal tuberosity
20 Metacarpal III (cannon bone)

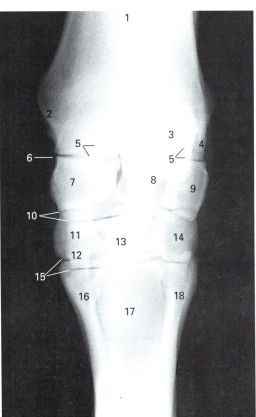

120. Radiograph of left carpal joint of horse, dorsopalmar projection.

1 Radius
2 Medial styloid process
3 Accessory carpal bone
4 Lateral styloid process
5 Trochlea of radius
6 Antebrachiocarpal joint
7 Radial carpal bone
8 Intermediate carpal bone
9 Ulnar carpal bone
10 Intercarpal joint
11 Second carpal bone
12 First carpal bone
13 Third carpal bone
14 Fourth carpal bone
15 Carpometacarpal joint
16 Metacarpal II (medial splint bone)
17 Metacarpal III (cannon bone)
18 Metacarpal IV (lateral splint bone)

121. Deep dissection of left carpus of horse, flexed dorsal view.

1 Radius
2 Groove for tendon of M. extensor carpi radialis
3 Groove for tendon of M. extensor digitorum lateralis
4 Facet on radius for articulation with radial carpal bone
5 Facet on radius for articulation with intermediate carpal bone
6 Facet on lateral styloid process for articulation with ulnar carpal bone
7 Medial collateral carpal ligament
8 Lateral collateral carpal ligament
9 Radial carpal bone
10 Dorsal intercarpal ligament between radial and intermediate carpal bones
11 Intermediate carpal bone
12 Dorsal intercarpal ligament between ulnar and intermediate carpal bones
13 Facet on ulnar carpal bone for articulation with fourth carpal bone
14 Facet on second carpal bone for articulation with radial carpal bone
15 Facet on third carpal bone for articulation with radial carpal bone
16 Facet on third carpal bone for articulation with intermediate carpal bone
17 Facet on fourth carpal bone for articulation with intermediate carpal bone
18 Facet on fourth carpal bone for articulation with ulnar carpal bone
19 Metacarpal tuberosity

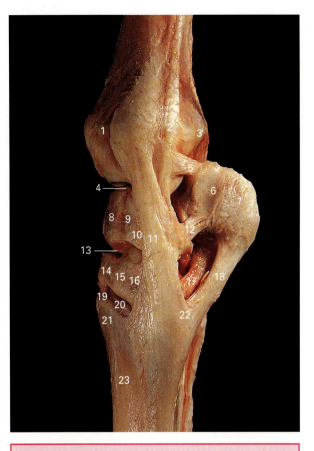

122. Deep dissection of left carpus of horse, lateral view.

1 Groove for tendon of
  M. extensor digitorum
  communis
2 Tendon of M. extensor
  digitorum lateralis
3 Transverse crest of radius
4 Antebrachiocarpal joint
5 Accessorioulnar ligament
6 Groove for tendon of
  M. ulnaris lateralis
7 Accessory carpal bone
8 Intermediate carpal bone
9 Dorsal intercarpal ligament
  between intermediate and
  ulnar carpal bones
10 Ulnar carpal bone
11 Lateral collateral carpal
   ligament
12 Accessoriocarpoulnar
   ligament

13 Intercarpal joint
14 Third carpal bone
15 Dorsal intercarpal
   ligament between third
   and fourth carpal bones
16 Fourth carpal bone
17 Accessorioquartal
   ligament
18 Accessoriometacarpal
   ligament
19 Dorsal carpometacarpal
   ligament
20 Carpometacarpal joint
21 Metacarpal tuberosity
22 Base of metacarpal IV
   (lateral splint bone)
23 Metacarpal III
   (cannon bone)

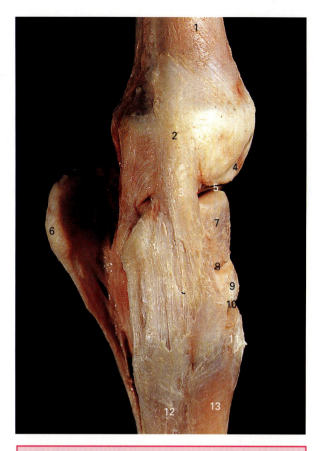

123. Deep dissection of left carpus of horse, medial view.

1 Radius
2 Medial styloid process
3 Medial collateral carpal
  ligament
4 Groove for tendon of M.
  abductor digiti I longus
5 Antebrachiocarpal joint
6 Accessory carpal bone
7 Radial carpal bone

8 Intercarpal joint
9 Third carpal bone
10 Carpometacarpal joint
11 Metacarpal tuberosity
12 Metacarpal II (medial
   splint bone)
13 Metacarpal III (cannon
   bone)

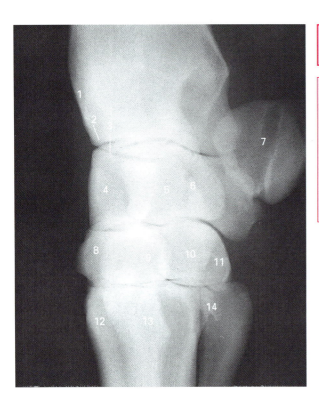

124. Radiograph of left carpal joint of horse, lateromedial projection.

1 Groove for tendon of M. extensor carpi radialis	8 Third carpal bone
2 Lateral border of medial articular surface	9 Second carpal bone
3 Medial border of medial articular surface	10 Fourth carpal bone
	11 First carpal bone
4 Radial carpal bone	12 Metacarpal III (cannon bone)
5 Intermediate carpal bone	13 Metacarpal II (medial splint bone)
6 Ulnar carpal bone	14 Metacarpal IV (lateral splint bone)
7 Accessory carpal bone	

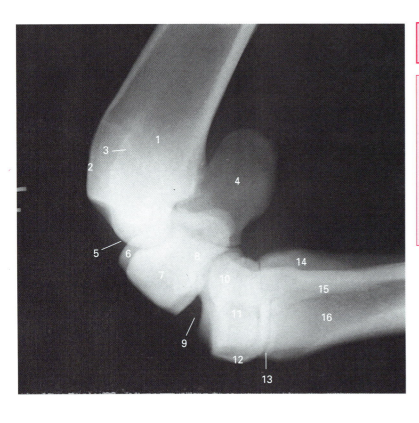

125. Radiograph of left carpal joint of horse, flexed lateromedial projection.

1 Radius	8 Ulnar carpal bone
2 Edge of groove for tendon of M. extensor carpi radialis	9 Intercarpal joint
	10 Second carpal bone
3 Edge of groove for tendon of M. extensor digitorum communis	11 Fourth carpal bone
	12 Third carpal bone
4 Accessory carpal bone	13 Carpometacarpal joint
5 Antebrachiocarpal joint	14 Metacarpal IV (lateral splint bone)
6 Intermediate carpal bone	15 Metacarpal II (medial splint bone)
7 Radial carpal bone	16 Metacarpal III (cannon bone)

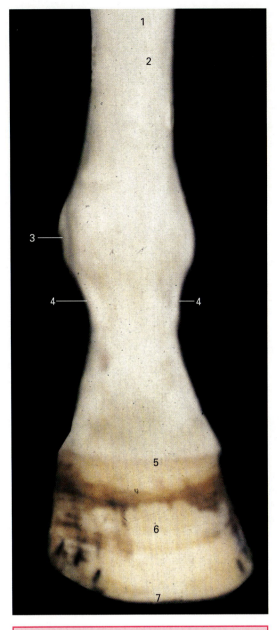

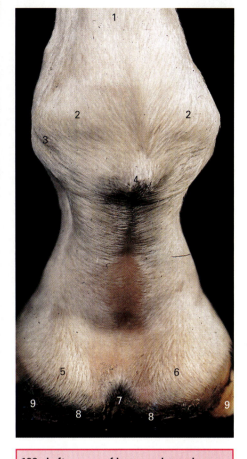

126. Left manus of horse, dorsal view.

127. Left manus of horse, lateral view.

128. Left manus of horse, palmar view.

1 Metacarpal region	4 Extensor branches
2 Tendon of M. extensor	of M. interosseus
digitorum communis	medius to tendon of
3 Level of	M. extensor
metacarpophalangeal	digitorum communis
(fetlock) joint	5 Coronet
	6 Wall of hoof
	7 Toe

1 Metacarpal III (cannon	6 Lateral extensor branch
bone)	of M. interosseus medius
2 Metacarpal IV (lateral	7 Ergot
splint bone)	8 Lateral cartilage of distal
3 M. interosseus medius	phalanx
(suspensory ligament)	9 Coronet
4 Tendons of M. flexor	10 Wall of hoof
digitorum superficialis and	11 Toe
M. flexor digitorum	12 Quarter
profundus	13 Heel
5 Level of	
metacarpophalangeal	
(fetlock) joint	

1 Metacarpal region	5 Lateral cartilage
2 Proximal	of distal phalanx
sesamoid bones	6 Medial cartilage
3 Level of	of distal phalanx
metacarpophalang	7 Cleft of frog
-eal (fetlock) joint	8 Bulbs of heel
4 Ergot	9 Hoof wall

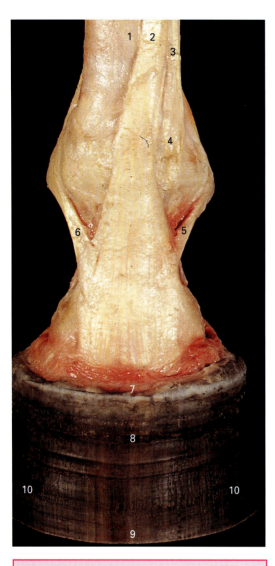

129. Superficial dissection of left manus of horse, dorsal view.

1 Metacarpal III (cannon bone)	5 Lateral extensor branch of M. interosseus medius
2 Tendon of M. extensor digitorum communis	6 Medial extensor branch of M. interosseus medius
3 Tendon of M. extensor digitorum lateralis	7 Coronet
4 Distal attachment of tendon of M. extensor digitorum lateralis	8 Wall of hoof
	9 Toe
	10 Quarters

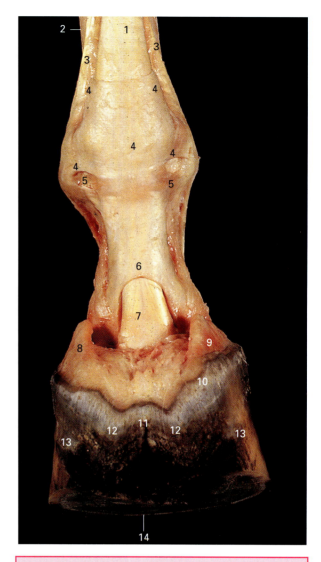

130. Superficial dissection of left manus of horse, palmar view.

1 Tendon of M. flexor digitorum superficialis	7 Tendon of M. flexor digitorum profundus
2 Metacarpal III (cannon bone)	8 Lateral cartilage of distal phalanx
3 M. interosseus medius (suspensory ligament)	9 Medial cartilage of distal phalanx
4 Superficial transverse metacarpal ligament (palmar annular ligament)	10 Coronet
	11 Cleft of frog
5 Vagina fibrosa (proximal digital annular ligament)	12 Bulbs of heel
	13 Wall of hoof
6 Manica flexoria	14 Sole of hoof

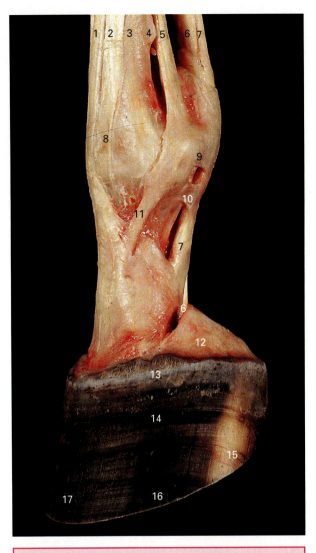

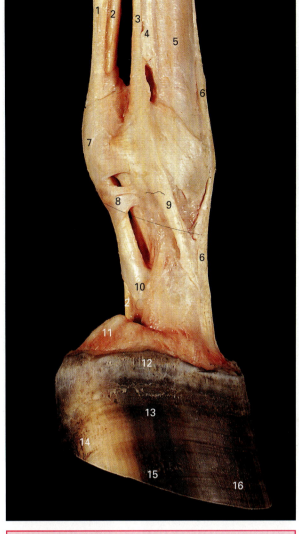

131. Superficial dissection of left manus of horse, lateral view.

132. Superficial dissection of left manus of horse, medial view.

1 Tendon of M. extensor digitorum communis	9 Superficial transverse metacarpal ligament (palmar annular ligament)
2 Tendon of M. extensor digitorum lateralis	10 Vagina fibrosa (proximal digital annular ligament)
3 Metacarpal III (cannon bone)	11 Lateral extensor branch of M. interosseus medius
4 Metacarpal IV (lateral splint bone)	12 Lateral cartilage of distal phalanx
5 M. interosseus medius (suspensory ligament)	13 Coronet
6 Tendon of M. flexor digitorum profundus	14 Wall of hoof
7 Tendon of M. flexor digitorum superficialis	15 Heel
8 Attachment of tendon of M. extensor digitorum lateralis	16 Quarter
	17 Toe

1 Tendon of M. flexor digitorum superficialis	8 Vagina fibrosa (proximal digital annular ligament)
2 Tendon of M. flexor digitorum profundus	9 Medial extensor branch of M. interosseus medius
3 M. interosseus medius (suspensory ligament)	10 Vagina fibrosa (distal digital annular ligament)
4 Metacarpal II (medial splint bone)	11 Medial cartilage of distal phalanx
5 Metacarpal III (cannon bone)	12 Coronet
6 Tendon of M. extensor digitorum communis	13 Wall of hoof
7 Superficial transverse metacarpal ligament (palmar annular ligament)	14 Heel
	15 Quarter
	16 Toe

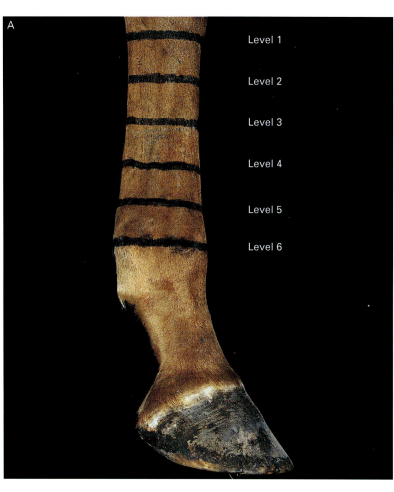

A

Level 1

Level 2

Level 3

Level 4

Level 5

Level 6

133. **Medial view of left manus of horse (A) showing six levels at which images were made using a 7.5 MHz ultrasound sector scanner with standoff pad (pictures B–G), and computerized tomography (pictures H–M). The leg was then sectioned at the six levels (pictures N–S).**

1 Metacarpal III (cannon bone)
2 Tendon of M. extensor digitorum communis
3 Interosseus metacarpal ligament between metacarpals II and III
4 Metacarpal II (medial splint bone)
5 Interosseus metacarpal ligament between metacarpals III and IV
6 Metacarpal IV (lateral splint bone)
7 Tendon of M. extensor digitorum lateralis
8 M. interosseus medius (suspensory ligament)
9 Medial extensor branch of M. interosseus medius
10 Lateral extensor branch of M. interosseus medius
11 Accessory ligament of M. flexor digitorum profundus (distal check ligament)
12 Medial palmar artery
13 Carpal sheath
14 Medial palmar digital artery
15 Lateral palmar digital artery
16 Medial proximal sesamoid bone
17 Lateral proximal sesamoid bone
18 Tendon of M. flexor digitorum profundus
19 Tendon of M. flexor digitorum superficialis

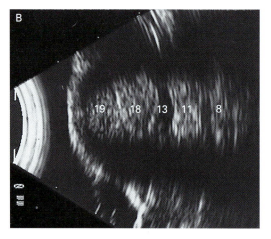

B

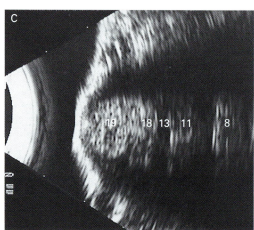

C

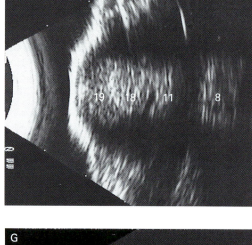

D

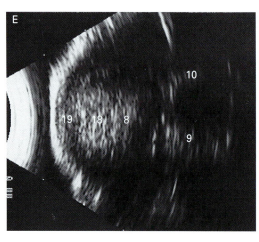

E

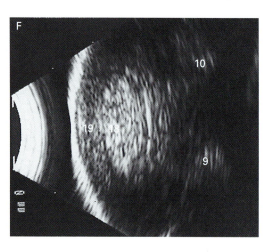

F

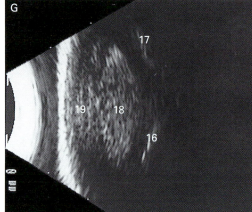

G

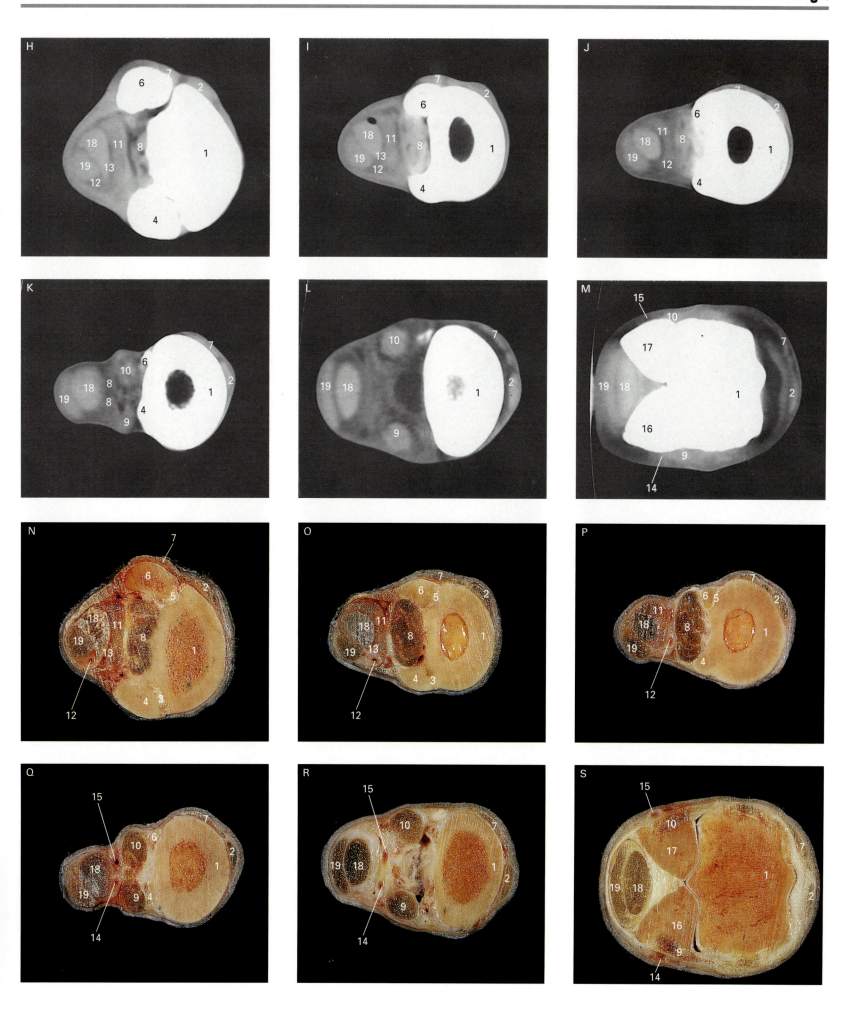

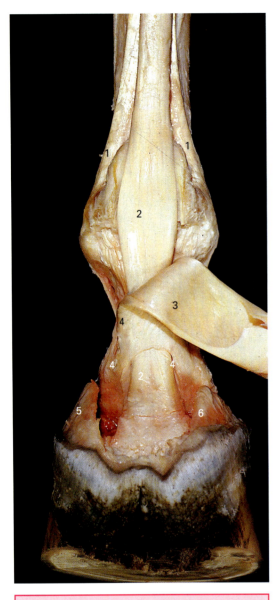

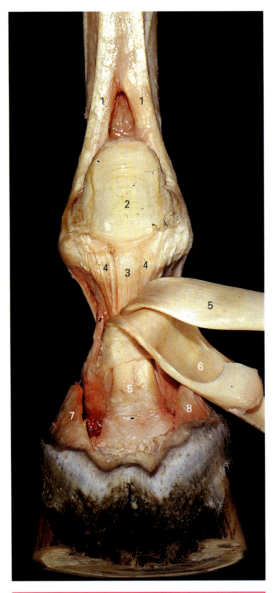

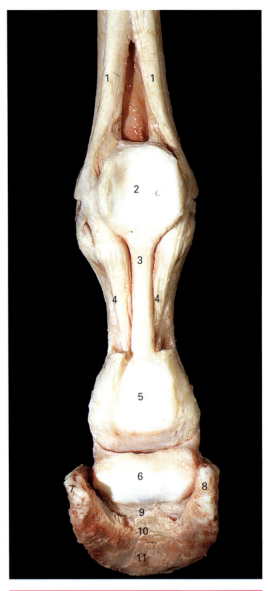

134. Deep dissection of left thoracic digit of horse, palmar view. The superficial transverse metacarpal ligament and the vagina fibrosa have been removed. The tendon of the M. flexor digitorum superficialis has been reflected.

1 Extensor branches of M. interosseus medius	4 Manica flexoria
2 Tendon of M. flexor digitorum profundus	5 Lateral cartilage of distal phalanx
3 Tendon of M. flexor digitorum superficialis (reflected)	6 Medial cartilage of distal phalanx

135. Deep dissection of left thoracic digit of horse, palmar view. The superficial transverse metacarpal ligament and the vagina fibrosa have been removed. The tendons of the M. flexor digitorum superficialis and M. flexor digitorum profundus have been reflected.

1 Extensor branches of M. interosseus medius	5 Tendon of M. flexor digitorum profundus
2 Palmar (intersesamoidean) ligament	6 Tendon of M. flexor digitorum superficialis
3 Straight sesamoidean ligament	7 Lateral cartilage of distal phalanx
4 Oblique sesamoidean ligament	8 Medial cartilage of distal phalanx

136. Deep dissection of left thoracic digit of horse, palmar view. The superficial transverse metacarpal ligament, vagina fibrosa, tendon of the M. flexor digitorum superficialis, and tendon of the M. flexor digitorum profundus have been removed. The wall, sole and frog of the hoof have been removed.

1 Extensor branches of M. interosseus medius	6 Flexor surface of distal sesamoid bone
2 Palmar (intersesamoidean) ligament	7 Lateral cartilage of distal phalanx
3 Straight sesamoidean ligament	8 Medial cartilage of distal phalanx
4 Oblique sesamoidean ligament	9 Flexor surface of distal phalanx
5 Fibrocartilaginous plate	10 Semilunar line
	11 Solar surface of distal phalanx

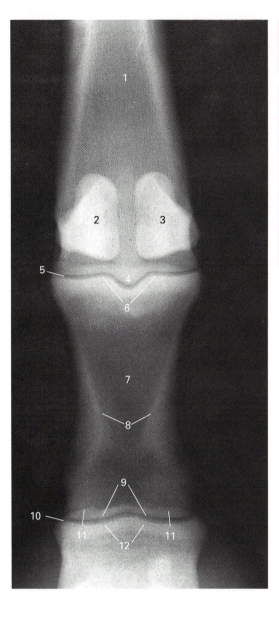

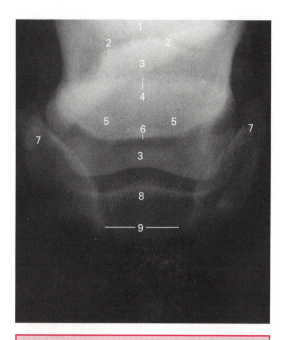

137. Radiograph of left metacarpophalangeal and proximal interphalangeal joints of horse, dorsopalmar projection.

1	Metacarpal III (cannon bone)	8	Ridges on palmar surface of proximal phalanx
2	Medial proximal sesamoid bone	9	Trochlea of proximal phalanx
3	Lateral proximal sesamoid bone	10	Proximal interphalangeal (pastern) joint
4	Sagittal ridge on trochlea of metacarpal III	11	Dorsal border of articular fovea of middle phalanx
5	Metacarpophalangeal joint (fetlock joint)	12	Palmar border of articular fovea of middle phalanx
6	Articular fovea of proximal phalanx		
7	Proximal phalanx		

139. Radiograph of distal manus of horse, dorsopalmar projection at 70° to the horizontal in the standing position.

1	Proximal phalanx	6	Distal border of distal sesamoid bone
2	Proximal interphalangeal (pastern) joint	7	Palmar process of distal phalanx
3	Middle phalanx	8	Extensor process of distal phalanx
4	Proximal border of distal sesamoid bone	9	Solar canal
5	Distal sesamoid (navicular) bone		

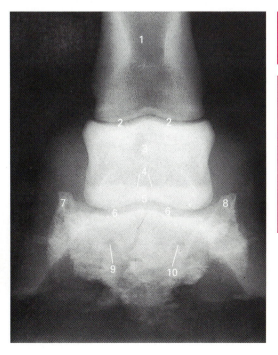

138. Radiograph of distal left digit of horse, dorsopalmar projection at 45° to the horizontal in the standing position.

1	Proximal phalanx	7	Medial palmar process
2	Proximal interphalangeal (pastern) joint	8	Lateral palmar process
3	Middle phalanx	9	Medial solar foramen
4	Extensor process of distal phalanx	10	Lateral solar foramen
5	Distal sesamoid (navicular) bone		
6	Distal interphalangeal (coffin) joint		

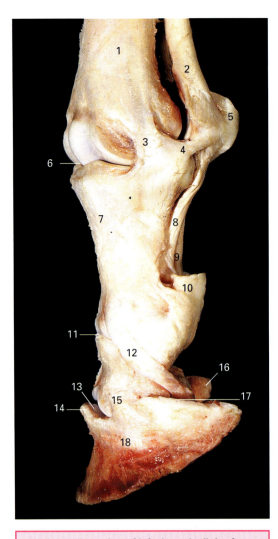

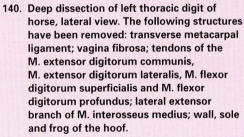

140. Deep dissection of left thoracic digit of horse, lateral view. The following structures have been removed: transverse metacarpal ligament; vagina fibrosa; tendons of the M. extensor digitorum communis, M. extensor digitorum lateralis, M. flexor digitorum superficialis and M. flexor digitorum profundus; lateral extensor branch of M. interosseus medius; wall, sole and frog of the hoof.

1 Metacarpal III (cannon bone)	11 Proximal interphalangeal (pastern) joint
2 M. interosseus medius (suspensory ligament)	12 Lateral collateral ligament of distal sesamoid bone (suspensory navicular ligament)
3 Lateral collateral metacarpophalangeal ligament	
4 Lateral collateral sesamoidean ligament	13 Distal interphalangeal (coffin) joint
5 Lateral proximal sesamoid bone	14 Extensor process of distal phalanx
6 Metacarpophalangeal (fetlock) joint	15 Lateral collateral ligament of distal interphalangeal joint
7 Proximal phalanx	
8 Oblique sesamoidean ligament	16 Medial process of distal phalanx
9 Straight sesamoidean ligament	17 Cut edge of lateral cartilage of distal phalanx
10 Cut edge of tendon of M. flexor digitorum superficialis	18 Distal phalanx (coffin bone)

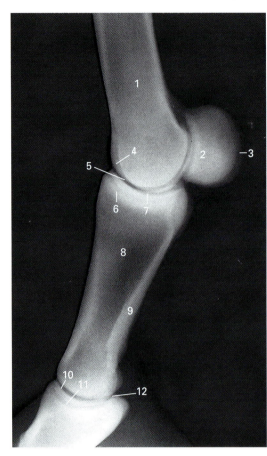

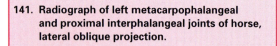

141. Radiograph of left metacarpophalangeal and proximal interphalangeal joints of horse, lateral oblique projection.

1 Metacarpal III (cannon bone)	7 Lateral border of articular fovea
2 Medial proximal sesamoid bone	8 Proximal phalanx
3 Lateral proximal sesamoid bone	9 Ridges on palmar surface of proximal phalanx
4 Sagittal ridge on trochlea of metacarpal III	10 Medial part of trochlea
5 Metacarpophalangeal (fetlock) joint	11 Lateral part of trochlea
6 Medial border of articular fovea	12 Proximal interphalangeal (pastern) joint

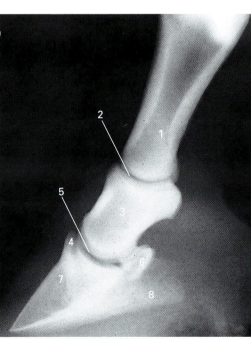

142. Radiograph of distal left digit of horse, lateromedial projection.

1 Proximal phalanx	5 Distal interphalangeal (coffin) joint
2 Proximal interphalangeal (pastern) joint	6 Distal sesamoid (navicular) bone
3 Middle phalanx	7 Distal phalanx (coffin bone)
4 Extensor process of distal phalanx	8 Palmar process of distal phalanx

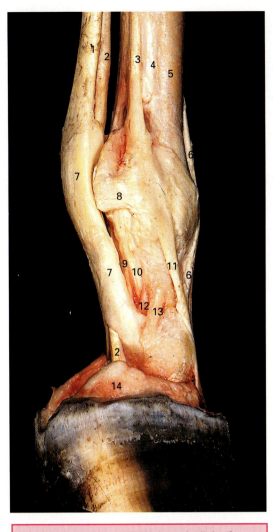

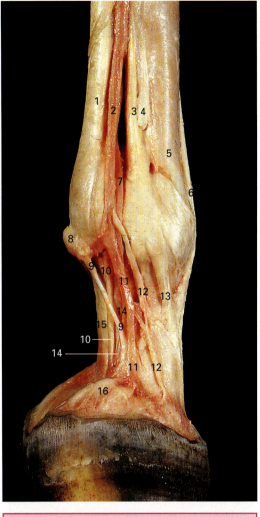

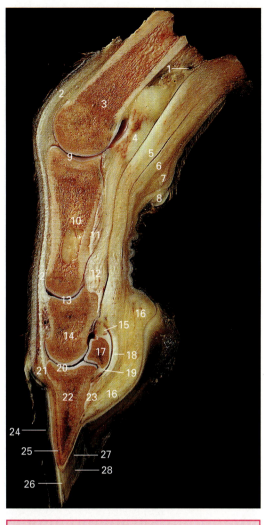

143. Deep dissection of left thoracic digit of horse, medial view. The superficial transverse metacarpal ligament and the vagina fibrosa have been removed.

1 Tendon of M. flexor digitorum superficialis	9 Straight sesamoidean ligament
2 Tendon of M. flexor digitorum profundus	10 Oblique sesamoidean ligament
3 M. interosseus medius (suspensory ligament)	11 Medial extensor branch of M. interosseus medius
4 Metacarpal II (medial splint bone)	12 Palmar ligament of proximal interphalangeal joint
5 Metacarpal III (cannon bone)	13 Medial collateral ligament of proximal interphalangeal joint
6 Tendon of M. extensor digitorum communis	14 Medial cartilage of distal phalanx
7 Manica flexoria	
8 Medial collateral sesamoidean ligament	

144. Dissection of nerves and vessels of distal left manus of horse, medial view.

1 Tendon of M. flexor digitorum superficialis	11 Medial palmar digital vein
2 Medial palmar vein	12 Dorsal branch of medial palmar digital nerve
3 M. interosseus medius (suspensory ligament)	13 Medial extensor branch of M. interosseus medius
4 Distal end of metacarpal II (button of medial splint bone)	14 Medial palmar digital artery
5 Metacarpal III (cannon bone)	15 Tendon of M. flexor digitorum profundus
6 Tendon of M. extensor digitorum communis	16 Medial cartilage of distal phalanx
7 Medial palmar artery	
8 Ergot	
9 Ligament of ergot	
10 Medial palmar digital nerve	

145. Median section through left thoracic digit of horse.

1 Proximal extent of digital synovial sheath	16 Digital cushion
2 Tendon of M. extensor digitorum communis	17 Distal sesamoid (navicular) bone
3 Metacarpal III (cannon bone)	18 Podotrochlear (navicular) bursa
4 Palmar ligament	19 Distal sesamoid impar ligament
5 Tendon of M. flexor digitorum profundus	20 Distal interphalangeal (coffin) joint
6 Tendon of M. flexor digitorum superficialis	21 Coronary corium
7 Fibrous tissue underlying ergot	22 Distal phalanx (coffin bone)
8 Ergot	23 Insertion of tendon of M. flexor digitorum profundus
9 Metacarpophalangeal (fetlock) joint	24 Wall of hoof
10 Proximal phalanx	25 Lamellae
11 Oblique sesamoidean ligament	26 White zone
12 Straight sesamoidean ligament	27 Sole corium
13 Proximal interphalangeal (pastern) joint	28 Sole of hoof
14 Middle phalanx	
15 Collateral sesamoidean (suspensory navicular) ligament	

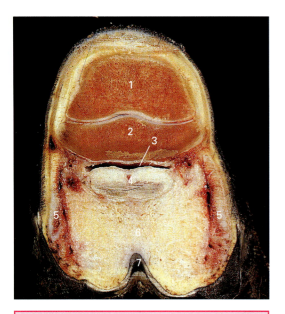

146. Frontal section of left hoof of horse, palmar view. Section is cut through the heels.

1 Middle phalanx	5 Cartilages of distal
2 Distal sesamoid	phalanx with
(navicular) bone	associated vascular
3 Podotrochlear	plexus
(navicular) bursa	6 Digital cushion
4 Tendon of M. flexor	7 Cleft of frog
digitorum profundus	

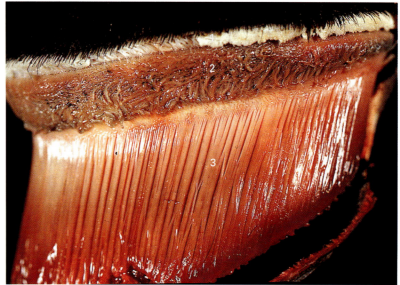

147. Corium of foot of horse, lateral view. The wall and epidermal lamellae have been removed.

1 Corium of periople	3 Lamellar corium
2 Coronary corium	(dermal lamellae)

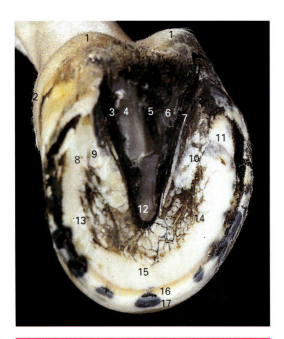

148. Left hoof of horse, solar view.

1 Bulbs of heel	10 Medial bar of hoof
2 Coronet	wall
3 Lateral paracuneal	11 Medial angle of sole
sulcus	12 Apex of frog
4 Lateral crus of frog	13 Lateral crus of sole
5 Central sulcus of frog	14 Medial crus of sole
6 Medial crus of frog	15 Central part of sole
7 Medial paracuneal	16 White zone
sulcus	17 Hoof wall (stratum
8 Lateral angle of sole	medium)
9 Lateral bar of hoof wall	

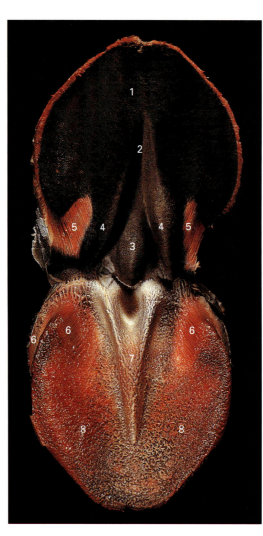

149. Foot of horse, solar view. The epidermal tissues have been reflected upwards. The wall and epidermal lamellae have been removed.

1 Dorsal surface of sole	6 Lamellar corium
2 Central furrow over	7 Corium of frog
apex of frog	8 Corium of sole
3 Spine of frog (frog stay)	
4 Junction of frog and	
bar	
5 Lamellae of bar	

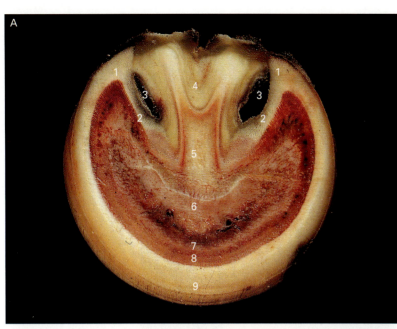

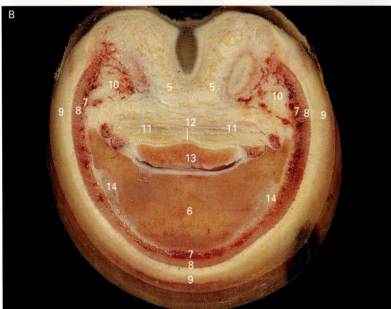

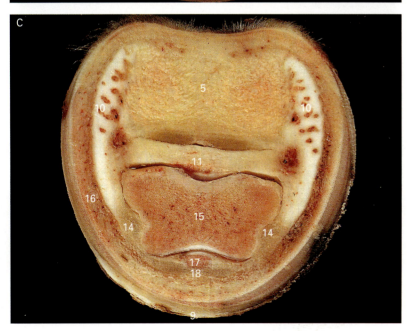

150. Transverse section through foot of horse, distal view. Sections are cut parallel to the coronary border: A, three fourths of the distance from the coronet to the distal border of the hoof wall; B, midway between the coronet and distal border of the hoof wall; C, just distal to the coronet.

1 Angle
2 Bar
3 Paracuneal sulcus
4 Frog
5 Digital cushion
6 Distal phalanx
7 Lamellar corium (dermal lamellae)
8 Lamellae of wall (epidermal lamellae)
9 Wall
10 Cartilage of distal phalanx and associated vascular plexus
11 Tendon of M. flexor digitorum profundus
12 Podotrochlear (navicular) bursa
13 Distal sesamoid (navicular) bone
14 Collateral ligament of distal interphalangeal joint
15 Middle phalanx
16 Coronary corium
17 Extensor process of distal phalanx
18 Tendon of M. extensor digitorum communis

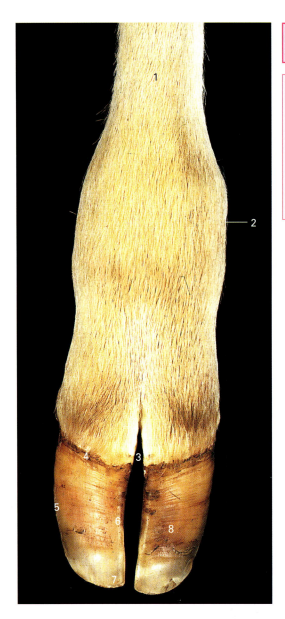

151. Left manus of ox, dorsal view.

1 Metacarpal region
2 Level of metacarpophalangeal joint
3 Interdigital cleft
4 Coronet, digit III
5 Abaxial hoof wall, digit III
6 Axial hoof wall, digit III
7 Toe of hoof, digit III
8 Digit IV

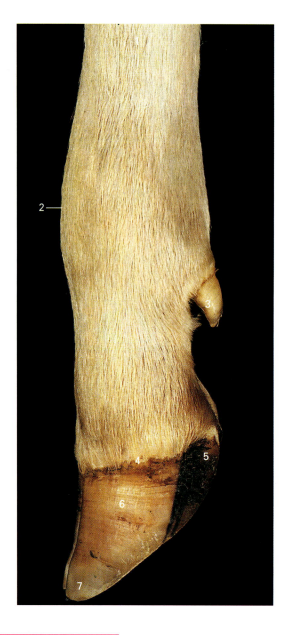

152. Left manus of ox, lateral view.

1 Metacarpal region
2 Level of metacarpophalangeal joint
3 Abaxial hoof wall, digit V
4 Coronet, digit IV
5 Bulb of heel, digit IV
6 Abaxial hoof wall, digit IV
7 Toe of hoof, digit IV

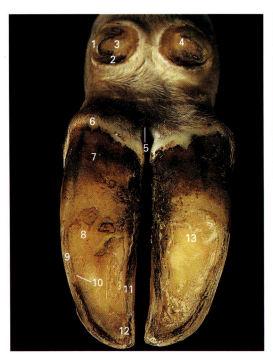

153. Left digits of ox, solar view.

1 Abaxial hoof wall, digit V
2 Axial hoof wall, digit V
3 Sole, digit V
4 Digit II
5 Interdigital cleft
6 Coronet, digit IV
7 Bulb of heel, digit IV
8 Sole of hoof, digit IV
9 Abaxial hoof wall, digit IV
10 White zone, digit IV
11 Axial hoof wall, digit IV
12 Toe of hoof, digit IV
13 Digit III

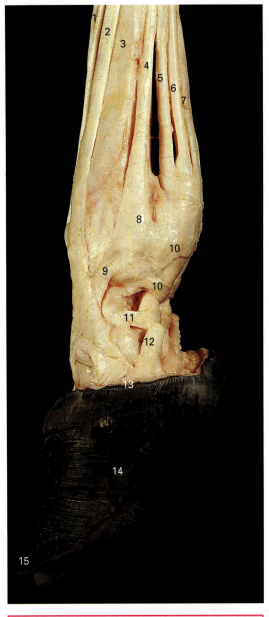

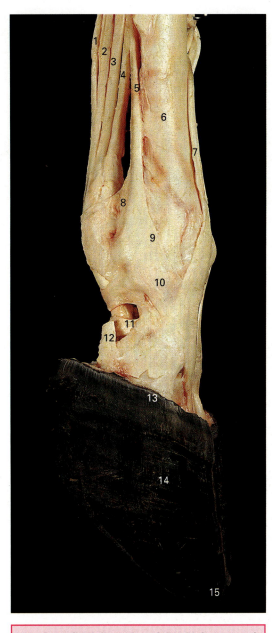

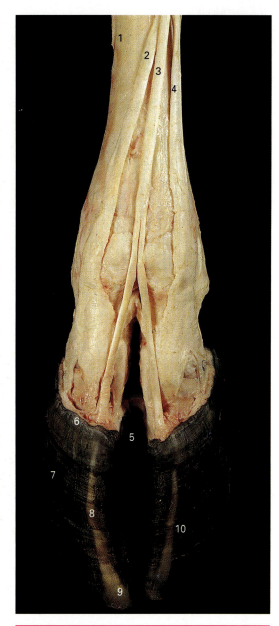

154. Superficial dissection of distal left manus of ox, lateral view. The accessory digits have been removed.

1 Tendon of M. extensor digitorum communis to digits III and IV	9 Abaxial branch of M. interosseus to tendon of M. extensor digitorum lateralis
2 Tendon of M. extensor digitorum lateralis	10 Superficial transverse metacarpal ligament (palmar annular ligament)
3 Metacarpals III and IV (fused)	11 Vagina fibrosa (proximal digital annular ligament)
4 M. interosseus (lateral abaxial tendon)	12 Distal ligament of accessory digit V
5 Tendon of M. interosseus to tendon of M. flexor digitorum superficialis	13 Coronet, digit IV
6 Tendon of M. flexor digitorum profundus	14 Abaxial hoof wall, digit IV
7 Tendon of M. flexor digitorum superficialis	15 Toe of hoof, digit IV
8 Attachment of M. interosseus to proximal sesamoid bone, digit IV	

155. Superficial dissection of distal left manus of ox, medial view. The accessory digits have been removed.

1 Tendon of M. flexor digitorum superficialis, superficial part	8 Superficial transverse metacarpal ligament (palmar annular ligament)
2 Tendon of M. flexor digitorum superficialis, deep part	9 Attachment of M. interosseus to sesamoid bone of digit III
3 Tendon of M. flexor digitorum profundus	10 Abaxial branch of M. interosseus to tendon of M. extensor digitorum communis
4 Tendon of M. interosseus to tendon of M. flexor digitorum superficialis	11 Vagina fibrosa (proximal digital annular ligament)
5 Tendon of M. interosseus (medial abaxial tendon)	12 Distal ligament of accessory digit II
6 Metacarpals III and IV (fused)	13 Coronet, digit III
7 Tendon of M. extensor digitorum communis to digit III	14 Abaxial hoof wall, digit III
	15 Toe of hoof, digit III

156. Superficial dissection of distal left manus of ox, dorsal view.

1 Metacarpals III and IV (fused)	5 Interdigital cleft
2 Tendon of M. extensor digitorum communis to digit III (M. extensor digitorum medialis)	6 Coronet, digit IV
	7 Abaxial hoof wall, digit IV
3 Tendon of M. extensor digitorum communis to digits III and IV	8 Axial hoof wall, digit IV
	9 Toe of hoof, digit IV
4 Tendon of M. extensor digitorum lateralis	10 Digit III

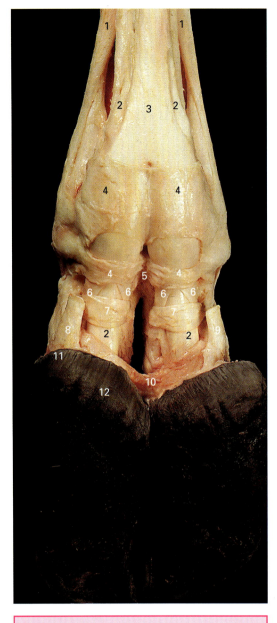

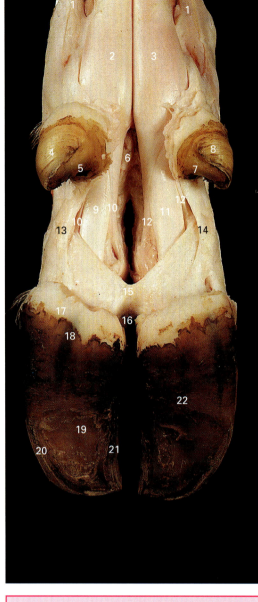

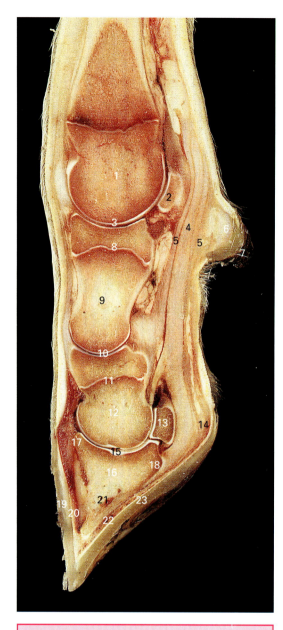

157. Superficial dissection of distal left manus of ox, palmar view. The accessory digits have been removed.

1 M. interosseus	7 Vagina fibrosa (proximal digital annular ligament)
2 Tendon of M. flexor digitorum profundus	8 Distal ligament of accessory digit V
3 Tendon of M. flexor digitorum superficialis	9 Distal ligament of accessory digit II
4 Superficial transverse metacarpal ligament (palmar annular ligament)	10 Distal interdigital ligament
5 Proximal interdigital ligament	11 Coronet, digit IV
6 Insertions of M. flexor digitorum superficialis	12 Bulb of heel, digit IV

158. Deep dissection of distal left manus of ox, palmar view. The superficial transverse metacarpal ligament and vagina fibrosa have been removed.

1 M. interosseus	11 Tendon of M. flexor digitorum profundus to digit III
2 Tendon of M. flexor digitorum superficialis to digit IV	12 Insertions of tendon of M. flexor digitorum superficialis to digit III
3 Tendon of M. flexor digitorum superficialis to digit III	13 Distal ligament of accessory digit V
4 Wall of hoof, digit V	14 Distal ligament of accessory digit II
5 Sole of hoof, digit V	15 Distal interdigital ligament
6 Proximal interdigital ligament	16 Interdigital cleft
7 Sole of hoof, digit II	17 Coronet, digit IV
8 Wall of hoof, digit II	18 Bulb of heel, digit IV
9 Tendon of M. flexor digitorum profundus to digit IV	19 Sole of hoof, digit IV
	20 Abaxial hoof wall, digit IV
10 Insertions of tendon of M. flexor digitorum superficialis to digit IV	21 Axial hoof wall, digit IV
	22 Digit III

159. Sagittal section through digit IV of left manus of immature ox.

1 Metacarpal III and IV (fused)	11 Proximal epiphysis of middle phalanx
2 Proximal sesamoid bone	12 Middle phalanx
3 Metacarpophalangeal joint	13 Distal sesamoid bone
4 Tendon of M. flexor digitorum profundus	14 Digital cushion
5 Manica flexoria	15 Distal interphalangeal joint
6 Phalanges of digit V	16 Distal phalanx, digit IV
7 Hoof of digit V	17 Extensor process
8 Proximal epiphysis of proximal phalanx	18 Flexor tuberosity
9 Proximal phalanx	19 Wall of hoof
10 Proximal interphalangeal joint	20 Lamellae
	21 Vessels in solar canal
	22 Corium of sole
	23 Sole of hoof

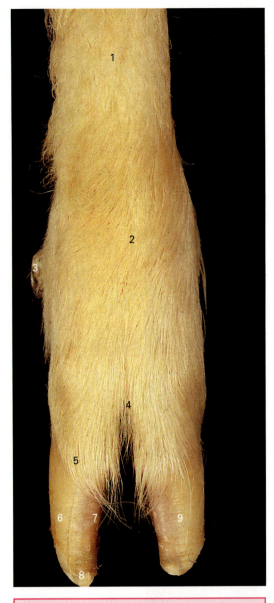

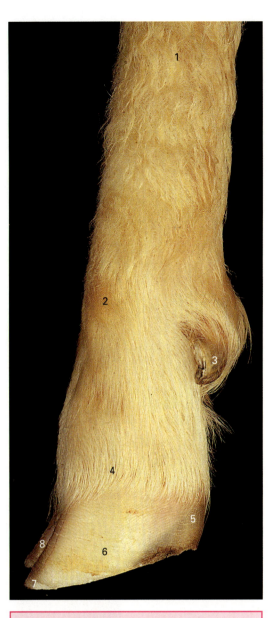

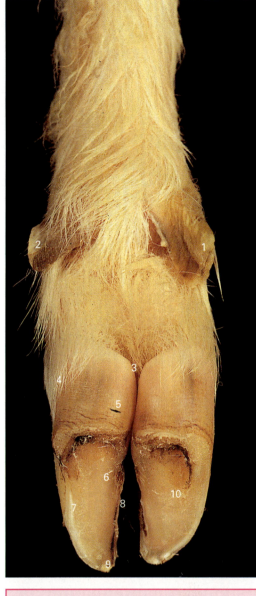

160. Left manus of sheep, dorsal view.

1 Metacarpal region	6 Abaxial hoof wall, digit III
2 Level of metacarpophalangeal joint	7 Axial hoof wall, digit III
3 Wall of hoof, digit II	8 Toe of hoof, digit III
4 Interdigital cleft	9 Digit IV
5 Coronet, digit III	

161. Left manus of sheep, lateral view.

1 Metacarpal region	4 Coronet, digit IV
2 Level of metacarpophalangeal joint	5 Bulb of heel, digit IV
3 Abaxial hoof wall, digit V	6 Abaxial hoof wall, digit IV
	7 Toe of hoof, digit IV
	8 Hoof wall, digit III

162. Left digits of sheep, solar view.

1 Digit V	7 Abaxial hoof wall, digit IV
2 Digit II	
3 Interdigital cleft	8 Axial hoof wall, digit IV
4 Coronet, digit IV	
5 Bulb of heel, digit IV	9 Toe of hoof, digit IV
6 Sole of hoof, digit IV	10 Digit III

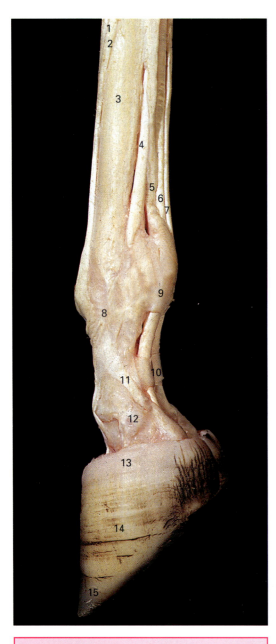

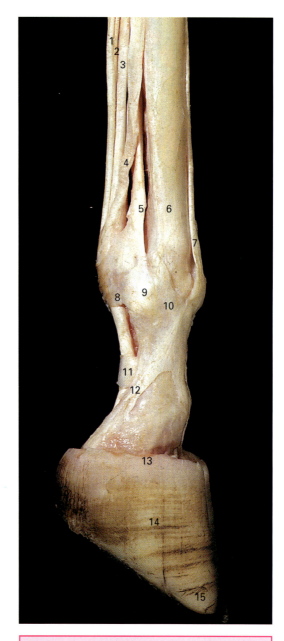

163. Superficial dissection of distal left manus of sheep, lateral view. The accessory digits have been removed.

1 Tendon of M. extensor digitorum communis to digits III and IV
2 Tendon of M. extensor digitorum lateralis
3 Metacarpals III and IV (fused)
4 M. interosseus
5 Branch of M. interosseus to tendon of M. flexor digitorum superficialis
6 Tendon of M. flexor digitorum profundus
7 Tendon of M. flexor digitorum superficialis
8 Abaxial branch of M. interosseus to extensor tendon of digit IV
9 Superficial transverse metacarpal ligament (palmar annular ligament)
10 Vagina fibrosa (proximal digital annular ligament)
11 Collateral sesamoidean ligament
12 Lateral collateral ligament of proximal interphalangeal joint, digit IV
13 Coronet, digit IV
14 Abaxial hoof wall, digit IV
15 Toe of hoof, digit IV

164. Superficial dissection of distal left manus of sheep, medial view. The accessory digits have been removed.

1 Tendon of M. flexor digitorum superficialis (superficial part)
2 Tendon of M. flexor digitorum superficialis (deep part)
3 Tendon of M. flexor digitorum profundus
4 Tendon of M. interosseus to tendon of M. flexor digitorum superficialis
5 Branch of M. interosseus to proximal sesamoid bone
6 Metacarpals III and IV (fused)
7 Tendon of M. extensor digitorum communis
8 Superficial transverse metacarpal ligament (palmar annular ligament)
9 Attachment of M. interosseus to proximal sesamoid bone
10 Abaxial branch of M. interosseus to extensor tendon of digit III
11 Vagina fibrosa (proximal digital annular ligament)
12 Collateral sesamoidean ligament
13 Coronet, digit III
14 Abaxial hoof wall, digit III
15 Toe of hoof, digit III

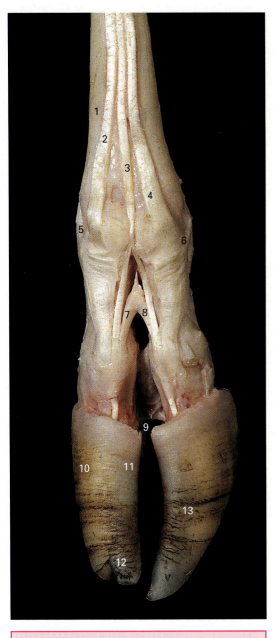

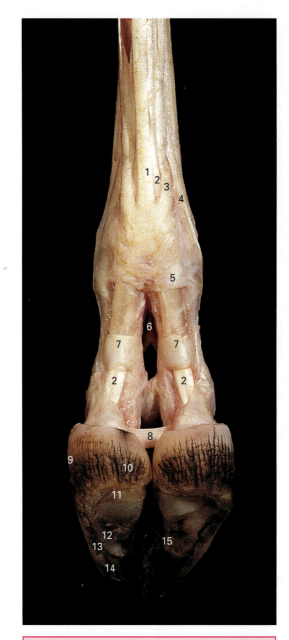

165. Superficial dissection of left manus of sheep, dorsal view.

166. Superficial dissection of left manus of sheep, palmar view. The accessory digits have been removed.

1 Metacarpals III and IV (fused)	7 Interdigital branch of M. interosseus to extensor tendon of digit III
2 Tendon of M. extensor digitorum communis to digit III	8 Interdigital branch of M. interosseus to extensor tendon of digit IV
3 Tendon of M. extensor digitorum communis to digits III and IV	9 Interdigital cleft
4 Tendon of M. extensor digitorum lateralis	10 Abaxial hoof wall, digit III
5 Abaxial branch of M. interosseus to extensor tendon of digit III	11 Axial hoof wall, digit III
6 Abaxial branch of M. interosseus to extensor tendon of digit IV	12 Toe of hoof, digit III
	13 Digit IV

1 Tendon of M. flexor digitorum superficialis	7 Vagina fibrosa (proximal digital annular ligament)
2 Tendon of M. flexor digitorum profundus	8 Distal interdigital ligament
3 Branch of M. interosseus to tendon of M. flexor digitorum superficialis	9 Abaxial part of bulb of heel, digit IV
4 Branch of M. interosseus to proximal sesamoid bone and extensor tendon of digit III	10 Axial part of bulb of heel, digit IV
	11 Solar part of bulb of heel, digit IV
5 Superficial transverse metacarpal ligament (palmar annular ligament)	12 Sole of hoof, digit IV
	13 White zone, digit IV
	14 Toe of hoof, digit IV
6 Proximal interdigital ligament	15 Digit III

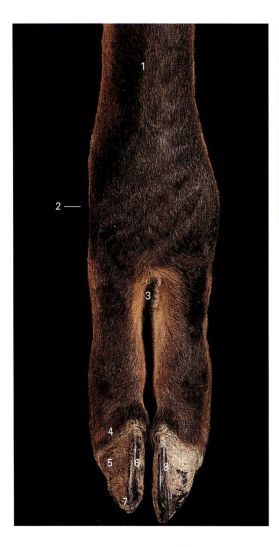

167. Left manus of llama, dorsal view.

1 Metacarpal region
2 Level of metacarpophalangeal joint
3 Interdigital cleft
4 Coronet, digit III
5 Abaxial hoof wall, digit III
6 Axial hoof wall, digit III
7 Toe of hoof, digit III
8 Digit IV

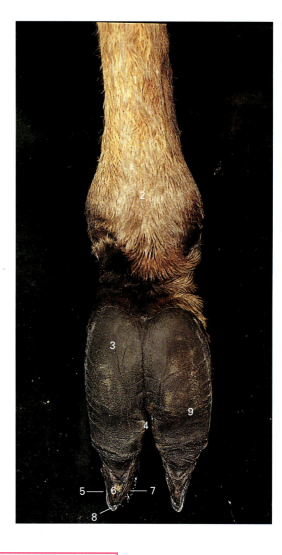

169. Left manus of llama, solar view.

1 Metacarpal region
2 Level of metacarpophalangeal joint
3 Digital pad, digit IV
4 Interdigital space
5 Abaxial hoof wall, digit IV
6 Sole of hoof, digit IV
7 Axial hoof wall, digit IV
8 Toe of hoof, digit IV
9 Digit III

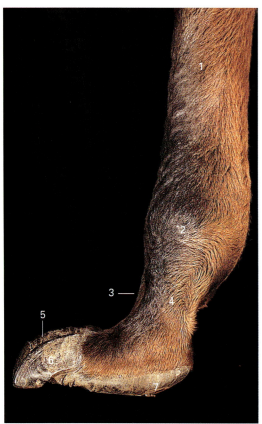

168. Left manus of llama, lateral view.

1 Metacarpal region
2 Level of metacarpophalangeal joint
3 Digit III
4 Digit IV
5 Hoof wall (slipper), digit III
6 Hoof wall (slipper), digit IV
7 Digital pad, digit IV

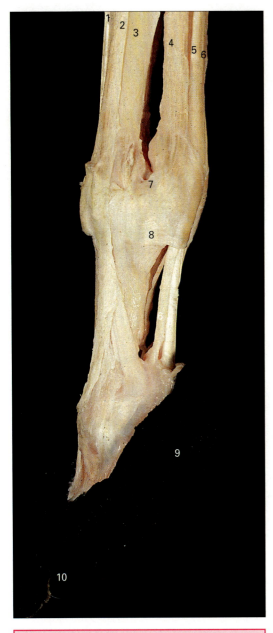

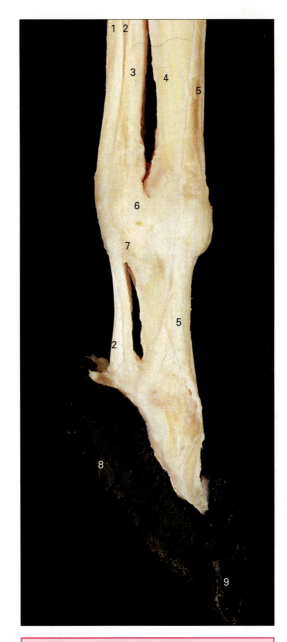

170. **Superficial dissection of distal left manus of llama, lateral view.**

171. **Superficial dissection of distal left manus of llama, medial view.**

1 Tendon of
  M. extensor digitorum
  communis
2 Tendon of
  M. extensor digitorum
  lateralis
3 Metacarpals III and IV
  (fused)
4 M. interosseus
5 Tendon of M. flexor
  digitorum profundus
6 Tendon of M. flexor
  digitorum superficialis
7 Attachment of
  M. interosseus to
  proximal sesamoid
  bone, digit IV
8 Superficial
  transverse
  metacarpal ligament
  (palmar annular
  ligament)
9 Digital pad, digit IV
10 Abaxial hoof wall,
  digit IV

1 Tendon of M. flexor
  digitorum superficialis
2 Tendon of M. flexor
  digitorum profundus
3 M. interosseus
4 Metacarpals III and IV
  (fused)
5 Tendon of M. extensor
  digitorum communis
6 Attachment of
  M. interosseus to
  proximal sesamoid
  bone, digit III
7 Superficial transverse
  metacarpal ligament
  (palmar annular
  ligament)
8 Digital pad, digit III
9 Abaxial hoof wall,
  digit III

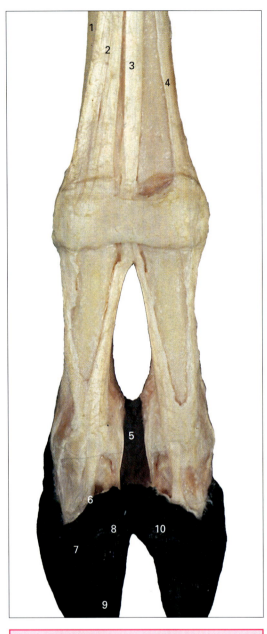

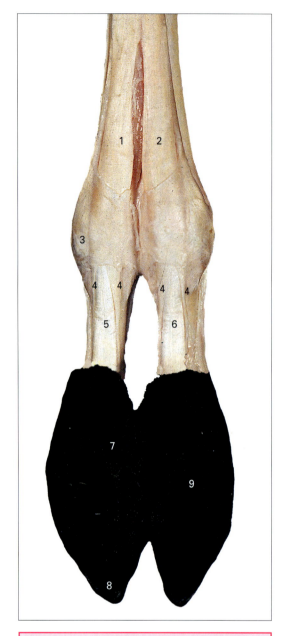

172. Superficial dissection of distal left manus of llama, dorsal view.

1 Metatarsals III and IV (fused)	5 Distal interdigital ligament
2 Tendon of M. extensor digitorum communis to digit III	6 Coronet, digit III
3 Tendon of M. extensor digitorum communis to digits III and IV	7 Abaxial hoof wall, digit III
4 Tendon of M. extensor digitorum lateralis	8 Axial hoof wall, digit III
	9 Toe of hoof, digit III
	10 Digit IV

173. Superficial dissection of distal left manus of llama, palmar view.

1 Tendon of M. flexor digitorum superficialis to digit IV	4 Manica flexoria
2 Tendon of M. flexor digitorum superficialis to digit III	5 Tendon of M. flexor digitorum profundus to digit IV
3 Superficial transverse metacarpal ligament (palmar annular ligament)	6 Tendon of M. flexor digitorum profundus to digit III
	7 Digital pad, digit IV
	8 Sole of hoof, digit IV
	9 Digit III

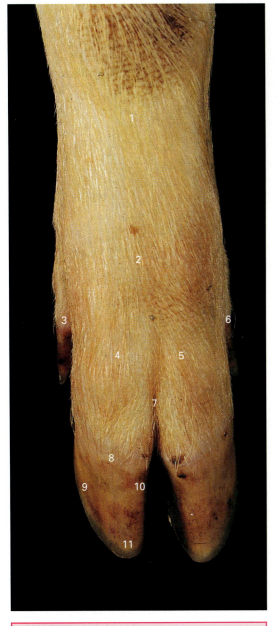

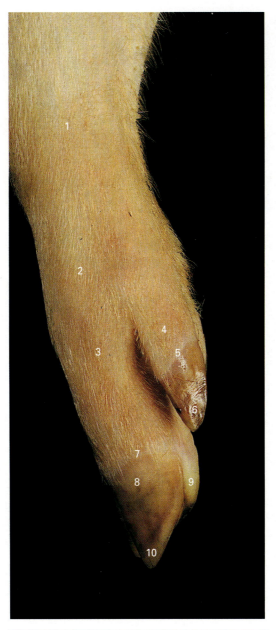

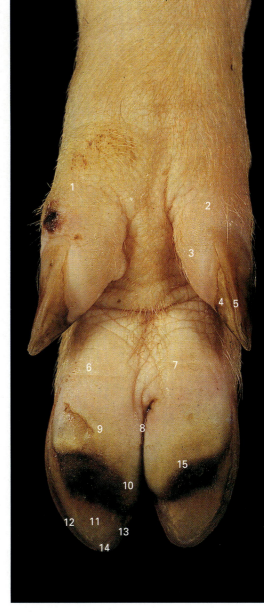

174. Left manus of pig, dorsal view.

1 Metacarpal region	7 Interdigital cleft
2 Level of metacarpophalangeal joint	8 Coronet, digit III
	9 Abaxial hoof wall, digit III
3 Digit II	10 Axial hoof wall, digit III
4 Digit III	11 Toe of hoof, digit III
5 Digit IV	
6 Digit V	

175. Left manus of pig, lateral view.

1 Metacarpal region	6 Abaxial hoof wall, digit V
2 Level of metacarpophalangeal joint	7 Coronet, digit IV
	8 Abaxial hoof wall, digit IV
3 Digit IV	9 Digital pad, digit IV
4 Digit V	10 Toe of hoof, digit IV
5 Coronet, digit V	

176. Left digits of pig, solar view.

1 Digit V	10 Apex of digital pad, digit IV
2 Digit II	
3 Digital pad, digit II	11 Sole of hoof, digit IV
4 Sole, digit II	12 Abaxial hoof wall, digit IV
5 Abaxial hoof wall, digit II	
6 Digit IV	13 Axial hoof wall, digit IV
7 Digit III	
8 Interdigital space	14 Toe of hoof, digit IV
9 Digital pad, digit IV	15 Digit III

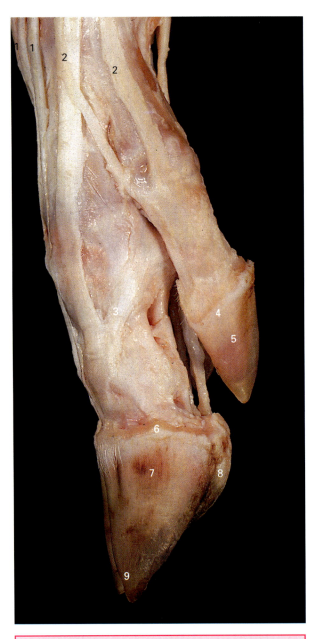

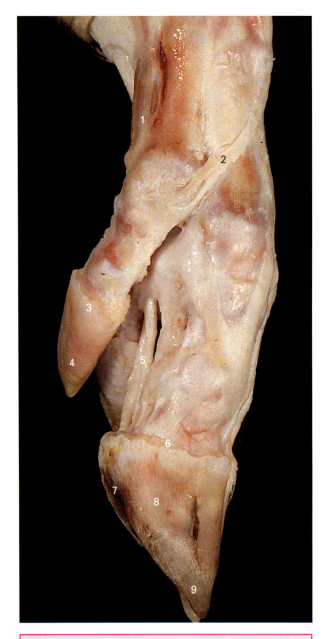

177. Superficial dissection of left distal manus of pig, lateral view.

1 Tendons of M. extensor digitorum communis	5 Abaxial hoof wall, digit V
2 Tendon of M. extensor digitorum lateralis	6 Coronet, digit IV
	7 Abaxial hoof wall, digit IV
3 Abaxial branch of M. interosseus to extensor tendon, digit IV	8 Digital pad, digit IV
	9 Toe of hoof, digit IV
4 Coronet, digit V	

178. Superficial dissection of left distal manus of pig, medial view.

1 M. abductor digiti II	6 Coronet, digit III
2 Tendon of M. extensor digitorum communis	7 Digital pad, digit III
	8 Abaxial hoof wall, digit III
3 Coronet, digit II	9 Toe of hoof, digit III
4 Abaxial hoof wall, digit II	
5 Tendon of M. flexor digitorum profundus to digit III	

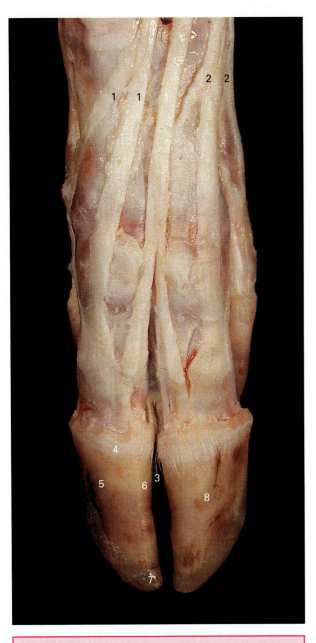

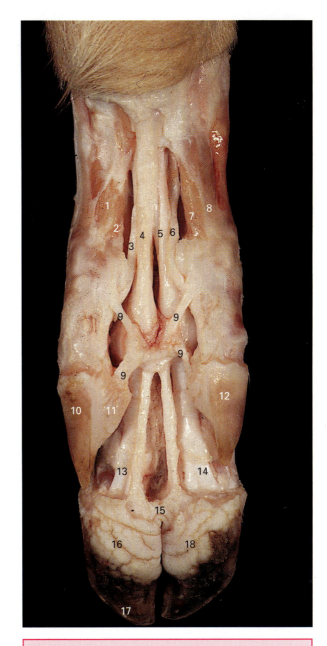

179. Superficial dissection of left distal manus of pig, dorsal view.

1 Tendons of M. extensor digitorum communis	4 Coronet, digit III
2 Tendons of M. extensor digitorum lateralis	5 Abaxial hoof wall, digit III
3 Interdigital cleft	6 Axial hoof wall, digit III
	7 Toe of hoof, digit III
	8 Digit IV

180. Superficial dissection of left distal manus of pig, palmar view.

1 M. abductor digiti V	10 Wall, digit V
2 M. flexor digiti V brevis	11 Digital pad, digit V
3 M. interosseus V	12 Wall, digit II
4 Tendon of M. flexor digitorum superficialis, superficial part	13 Tendon of M. flexor digitorum profundus to digit IV
5 Tendon of M. flexor digitorum superficialis, deep part	14 Tendon of M. flexor digitorum profundus to digit III
6 Tendon of M. flexor digitorum profundus to digit II	15 Distal interdigital ligament
7 M. lumbricales II	16 Digital pad, digit IV
8 M. abductor digiti II	17 Sole, digit IV
9 Deep transverse metacarpal ligaments	18 Digit III

5 Pelvic Limb

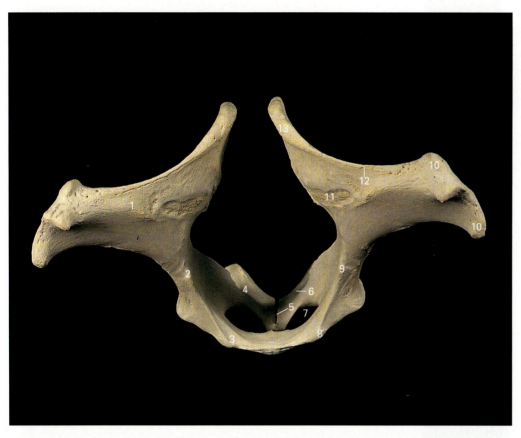

181. Ossa coxarum of horse, craniodorsal view.

1	Wing of ilium	8	Pubic tubercle
2	Body of ilium	9	Arcuate (iliopectineal)
3	Pubis		line
4	Ischium	10	Coxal tuberosity
5	Pelvic symphysis, ischiatic	11	Auricular surface
	part	12	Iliac crest
6	Ischiatic arch	13	Sacral tuberosity
7	Obturator foramen		

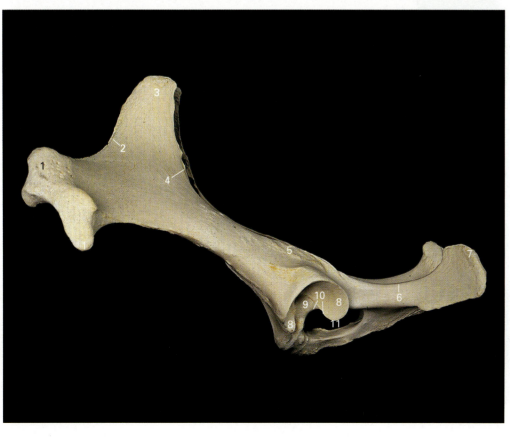

182. Ossa coxarum of horse, left lateral view.

1	Coxal tuberosity	7	Ischiatic tuberosity
2	Crest of ilium	8	Articular surface of
3	Sacral tuberosity		acetabulum
4	Greater ischiatic notch	9	Acetabular fossa
5	Ischiatic spine	10	Acetabular notch
6	Lesser ischiatic notch	11	Obturator foramen

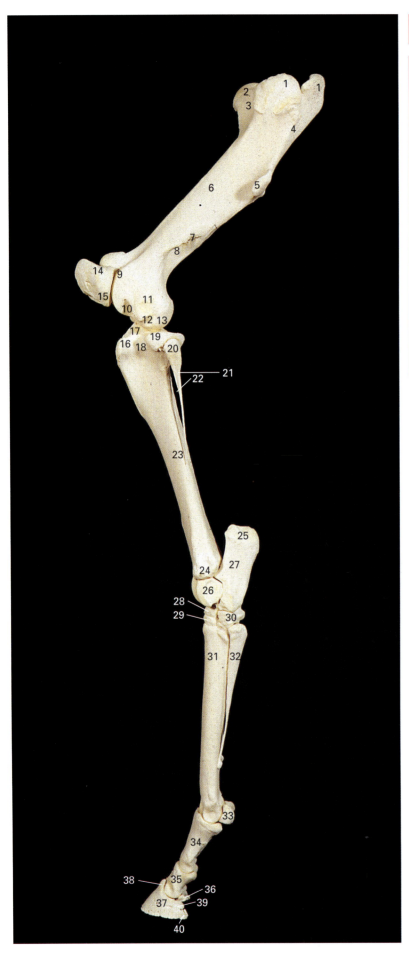

Femur
1 Greater trochanter
2 Head
3 Neck
4 Intertrochanteric crest
5 Third trochanter
6 Body
7 Lateral supracondylar
   tuberosity
8 Supracondylar fossa
9 Trochlea
10 Extensor fossa
11 Lateral epicondyle
12 Popliteal fossa
13 Lateral condyle

Patella
14 Base
15 Apex

Crus
16 Tibial tuberosity
17 Intercondylar eminence
18 Extensor sulcus
19 Lateral condyle
20 Head of fibula

21 Body of fibula
22 Interosseous space
23 Body of tibia
24 Lateral malleolus

Pes
25 Calcaneal tuber
26 Talus
27 Calcaneus
28 Central tarsal bone
29 Third tarsal bone
30 Fourth tarsal bone
31 Metatarsal III (cannon
    bone)
32 Metatarsal IV (lateral
    splint bone)
33 Proximal sesamoid bone
34 Proximal phalanx
35 Middle phalanx
36 Distal sesamoid
    (navicular) bone
37 Distal phalanx (coffin
    bone)
38 Extensor process
39 Lateral parietal sulcus
40 Lateral process

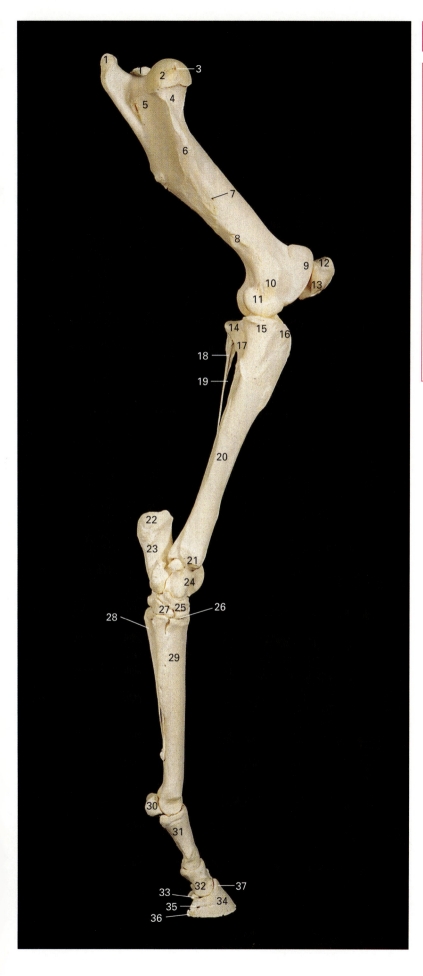

184. Skeleton of left pelvic limb of horse, medial view.

Femur
1 Greater trochanter
2 Head
3 Fovea
4 Neck
5 Trochanteric fossa
6 Lesser trochanter
7 Nutrient foramen
8 Medial supracondyloid tuberosity
9 Trochlea
10 Medial epicondyle
11 Medial condyle

Patella
12 Base
13 Apex

Crus
14 Lateral condyle
15 Medial condyle
16 Tibial tuberosity
17 Popliteal notch
18 Fibula
19 Interosseous space

20 Body of tibia
21 Medial malleolus

Pes
22 Calcaneal tuber
23 Calcaneus
24 Talus
25 Central tarsal bone
26 Third tarsal bone
27 First and second tarsal bones (fused)
28 Metatarsal II (medial splint bone)
29 Metatarsal III (cannon bone)
30 Proximal sesamoid bone
31 Proximal phalanx
32 Middle phalanx
33 Distal sesamoid (navicular) bone
34 Distal phalanx (coffin bone)
35 Medial parietal sulcus
36 Medial process
37 Extensor process

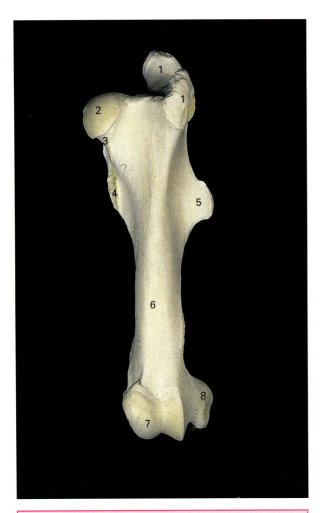

185. Left femur of horse, cranial view

1 Greater trochanter	5 Third trochanter
2 Head	6 Body
3 Neck	7 Trochlea
4 Lesser trochanter	8 Lateral epicondyle

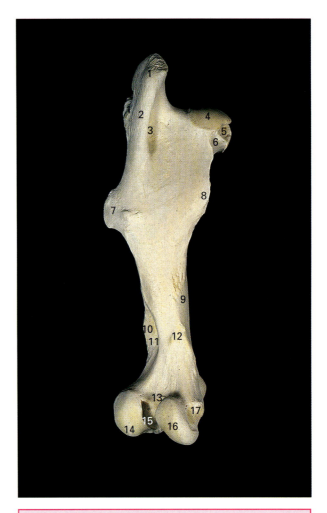

186. Left femur of horse, caudal view.

1 Greater trochanter	10 Lateral supracondyloid
2 Intertrochanteric crest	tuberosity
3 Trochanteric fossa	11 Supracondyloid fossa
4 Head	12 Medial supracondyloid
5 Fovea	tuberosity
6 Neck	13 Intercondylar line
7 Third trochanter	14 Lateral condyle
8 Lesser trochanter	15 Intercondylar fossa
9 Groove for femoral vessels	16 Medial condyle
	17 Medial epicondyle

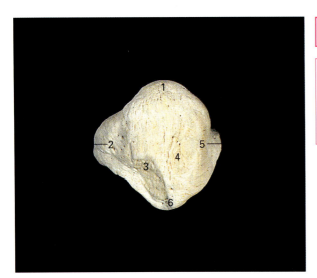

187. Left patella of horse, cranial view.

1 Base	4 Attachment area of lateral
2 Medial border	patellar ligament
3 Attachment area of middle	5 Lateral border
patellar ligament	6 Apex

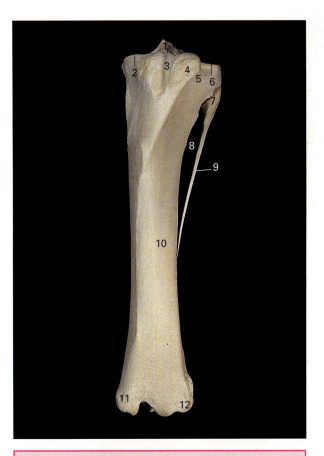

188. Left tibia and fibula of horse, cranial view.

1 Intercondylar eminence	7 Head of fibula
2 Medial condyle	8 Interosseous space
3 Groove for middle patellar ligament	9 Body of fibula
4 Tibial tuberosity	10 Body of tibia
5 Extensor sulcus	11 Medial malleolus
6 Lateral condyle	12 Lateral malleolus

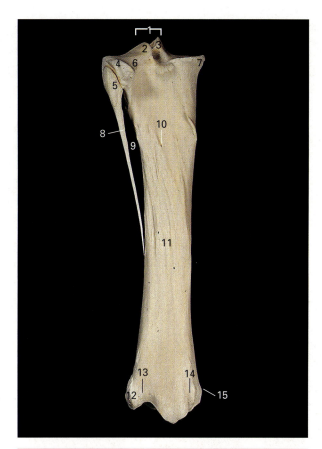

189. Left tibia and fibula of horse, caudal view.

1 Intercondylar eminence	9 Interosseous space
2 Lateral intercondylar tubercle	10 Nutrient foramen
3 Medial intercondylar tubercle	11 Body of tibia
4 Lateral condyle	12 Lateral malleolus
5 Head of fibula	13 Groove for tendon of M. extensor digitorum lateralis
6 Popliteal notch	14 Groove for tendon of M. flexor digitorum longus
7 Medial condyle	15 Medial malleolus
8 Body of fibula	

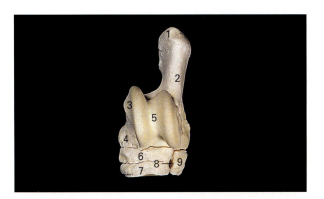

190 Left tarsal bones of horse, dorsal view.

1 Calcaneal tuber	7 Third tarsal bone
2 Calcaneus	8 Vascular canal
3 Talus	9 Fourth tarsal bone
4 Distal tuberosity of talus	
5 Trochlea	
6 Central tarsal bone	

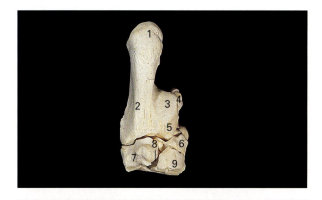

191. Left tarsal bones of horse, plantar view.

1 Calcaneal tuber	5 Sustentaculum tali
2 Calcaneus	6 Central tarsal bone
3 Tarsal groove for tendon of M. flexor digitorum profundus	7 Fourth tarsal bone
	8 Vascular canal
4 Talus	9 First and second tarsal bones (fused)

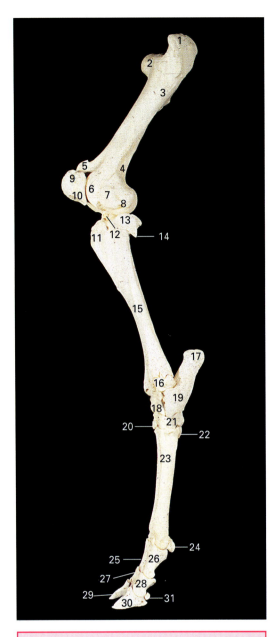

192. Skeleton of left pelvic limb of ox, lateral view.

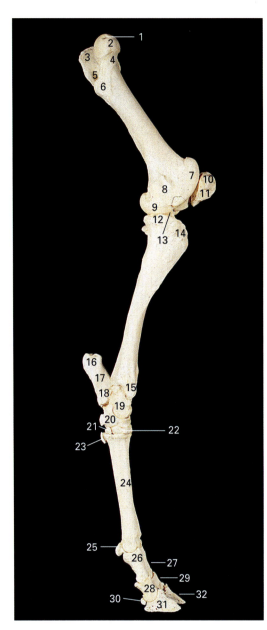

193. Skeleton of left pelvic limb of ox, medial view.

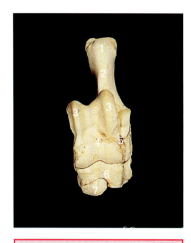

194. Left tarsal bones of ox, dorsal view.

1 Calcaneal tuber	6 Centroquartal bone
2 Calcaneus	7 Second and third tarsal bones (fused)
3 Trochlea	
4 Talus	
5 Tarsal sinus	

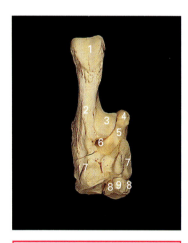

195. Left tarsal bones of ox, plantar view.

1 Calcaneal tuber	7 Centroquartal bone
2 Calcaneus	8 Second and third tarsal bones (fused)
3 Sustentaculum tali	9 First tarsal bone
4 Trochlea	
5 Talus	
6 Tarsal sinus	

Figure 192 key

Femur
1 Greater trochanter
2 Head
3 Third trochanter
4 Supracondyloid fossa
5 Medial crest of trochlea
6 Lateral crest of trochlea
7 Lateral epicondyle
8 Lateral condyle

Patella
9 Base
10 Apex

Crus
11 Tibial tuberosity
12 Intercondylar eminence
13 Lateral condyle
14 Head of fibula
15 Body of tibia
16 Lateral malleolus

Pes
17 Calcaneal tuber
18 Talus
19 Calcaneus
20 Second and third tarsal bones (fused)
21 Centroquartal bone
22 Metatarsal sesamoid bone
23 Metatarsals III and IV (fused)
24 Proximal sesamoid bone, digit IV
25 Proximal phalanx, digit III
26 Proximal phalanx, digit IV
27 Middle phalanx, digit III
28 Middle phalanx, digit IV
29 Distal phalanx, digit III
30 Distal phalanx, digit IV
31 Distal sesamoid bone, digit IV

Figure 193 key

Femur
1 Fovea
2 Head
3 Greater trochanter
4 Neck
5 Trochanteric fossa
6 Lesser trochanter
7 Trochlea
8 Medial epicondyle
9 Medial condyle

Patella
10 Base
11 Apex

Crus
12 Medial condyle of tibia
13 Intercondylar eminence
14 Tibial tuberosity
15 Medial malleolus

Pes
16 Calcaneal tuber
17 Calcaneus
18 Sustentaculum tali
19 Talus
20 Centroquartal bone
21 First tarsal bone
22 Second and third tarsal bones (fused)
23 Metatarsal sesamoid bone
24 Metatarsals III and IV (fused)
25 Proximal sesamoid bone, digit III
26 Proximal phalanx, digit III
27 Proximal phalanx, digit IV
28 Middle phalanx, digit III
29 Middle phalanx, digit IV
30 Distal sesamoid bone, digit III
31 Distal phalanx, digit III
32 Distal phalanx, digit IV

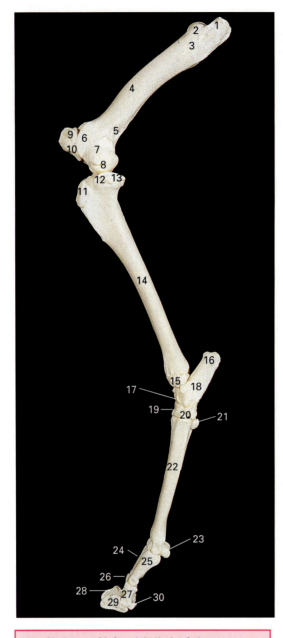

196. Skeleton of left pelvic limb of sheep, lateral view.

196. Skeleton of left pelvic limb of sheep, lateral view.

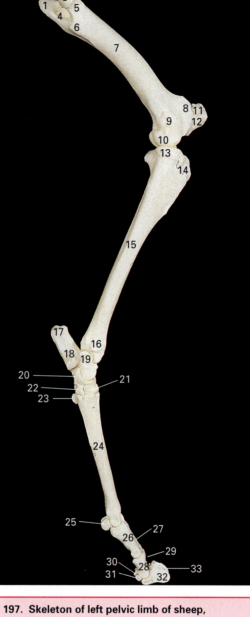

197. Skeleton of left pelvic limb of sheep, medial view.

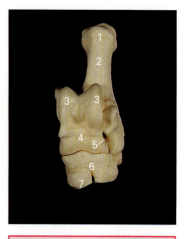

198. Left tarsal bones of sheep, dorsal view.

1	Calcaneal tuber	6	Centroquartal bone
2	Calcaneus	7	Second and third tarsal bones (fused)
3	Trochlea		
4	Talus		
5	Tarsal sinus		

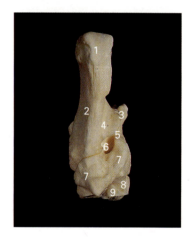

199. Left tarsal bones of sheep, plantar view.

1	Calcaneal tuber	7	Centroquartal bone
2	Calcaneus	8	Second and third tarsal bones (fused)
3	Sustentaculum tali	9	First tarsal bone
4	Trochlea		
5	Talus		
6	Tarsal sinus		

Femur
1 Greater trochanter
2 Head
3 Third trochanter
4 Body
5 Supracondyloid fossa
6 Trochlea
7 Lateral epicondyle
8 Lateral condyle

Patella
9 Base
10 Apex

Crus
11 Tibial tuberosity
12 Lateral condyle
13 Head of fibula
14 Body of tibia
15 Lateral malleolus

Pes
16 Calcaneal tuber
17 Talus
18 Calcaneus
19 Second and third tarsal bones (fused)

20 Centroquartal bone
21 Metatarsal sesamoid bone
22 Metatarsals III and IV (fused)
23 Proximal sesamoid bone, digit IV
24 Proximal phalanx, digit III
25 Proximal phalanx, digit IV
26 Middle phalanx, digit III
27 Middle phalanx, digit IV
28 Distal phalanx, digit III
29 Distal phalanx, digit IV
30 Distal sesamoid bone, digit IV

Femur
1 Greater trochanter
2 Fovea
3 Head
4 Trochanteric fossa
5 Neck
6 Lesser trochanter
7 Body
8 Trochlea
9 Medial epicondyle
10 Medial condyle

Patella
11 Base
12 Apex

Crus
13 Medial condyle of tibia
14 Tibial tuberosity
15 Body of tibia
16 Medial malleolus

Pes
17 Calcaneal tuber
18 Calcaneus
19 Talus
20 Centroquartal bone

21 Second and third tarsal bones (fused)
22 First tarsal bone
23 Metatarsal sesamoid bone
24 Metatarsals III and IV (fused)
25 Proximal sesamoid bone, digit III
26 Proximal phalanx, digit III
27 Proximal phalanx, digit IV
28 Middle phalanx, digit III
29 Middle phalanx, digit IV
30 Distal sesamoid bone, digit IV
31 Distal sesamoid bone, digit III
32 Distal phalanx, digit III
33 Distal phalanx, digit IV

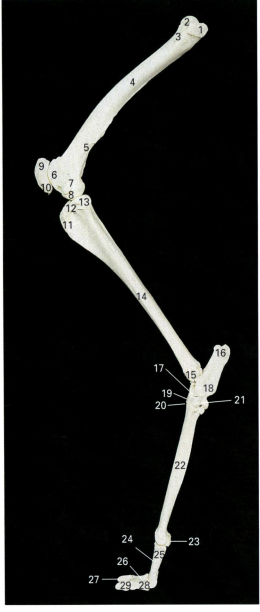

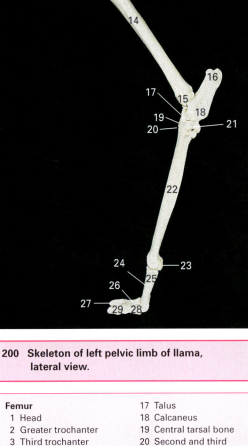

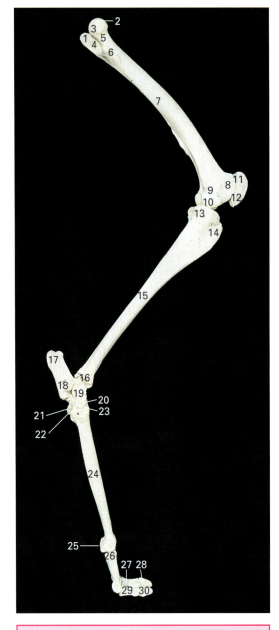

201. Skeleton of left pelvic limb of llama, medial view.

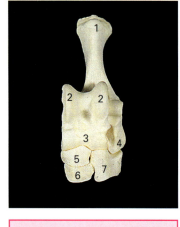

202. Left tarsal bones of llama, dorsal view.

1	Calcaneal	6	Second
	tuber		and third
2	Trochlea		tarsal bones
3	Talus		(fused)
4	Calcaneus	7	Fourth
5	Central tarsal		tarsal
	bone		bone

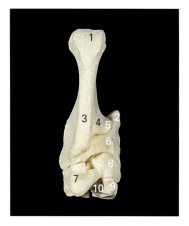

203. Left tarsal bones of llama, plantar view.

Femur
1 Head
2 Greater trochanter
3 Third trochanter
4 Body
5 Supracondyloid fossa
6 Trochlea
7 Lateral epicondyle
8 Lateral condyle

Patella
9 Base
10 Apex

Crus
11 Tibial tuberosity
12 Lateral condyle
13 Head of fibula
14 Body of tibia
15 Lateral malleolus

Pes
16 Calcaneal tuber

17 Talus
18 Calcaneus
19 Central tarsal bone
20 Second and third tarsal bones (fused)
21 Fourth tarsal bone
22 Metatarsals III and IV (fused)
23 Proximal sesamoid bone, digit IV
24 Proximal phalanx, digit III
25 Proximal phalanx, digit V
26 Middle phalanx, digit III
27 Distal phalanx, digit III
28 Middle phalanx, digit IV
29 Distal phalanx, digit IV

Femur
1 Greater trochanter
2 Fovea
3 Head
4 Trochanteric fossa
5 Neck
6 Lesser trochanter
7 Body
8 Trochlea
9 Medial epicondyle
10 Medial condyle

Patella
11 Base
12 Apex

Crus
13 Medial condyle of tibia
14 Tibial tuberosity
15 Body of tibia
16 Medial malleolus

Pes
17 Calcaneal tuber
18 Calcaneus
19 Talus
20 Central tarsal bone
21 Fourth tarsal bone
22 First tarsal bone
23 Second and third tarsal bones (fused)
24 Metatarsals III and IV (fused)
25 Proximal sesamoid bone, digit III
26 Proximal phalanx, digit III
27 Middle phalanx, digit IV
28 Distal phalanx, digit IV
29 Middle phalanx, digit III
30 Distal phalanx, digit III

1	Calcaneal	6	Talus
	tuber	7	Fourth tarsal
2	Trochlea		bone
3	Calcaneus	8	Central tarsal
4	Groove for		bone
	tendon of M.	9	First tarsal
	flexor		bone
	digitorum	10	Second and
	profundus		third tarsal
5	Sustentaculum		bones
	tali		(fused)

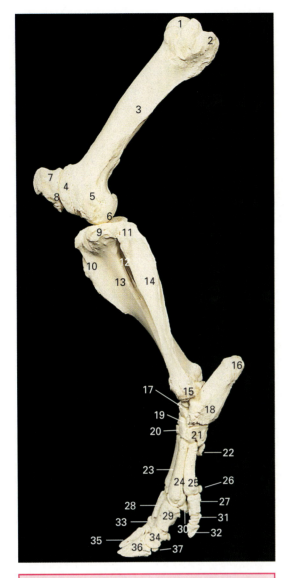

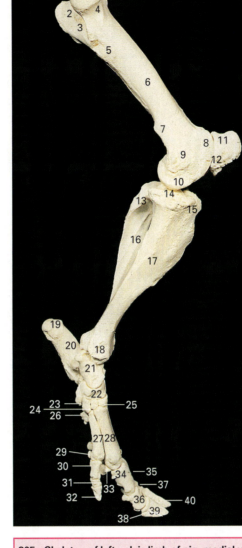

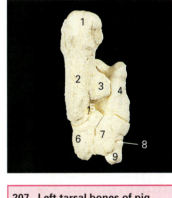

206. Left tarsal bones of pig, dorsal view.

1	Calcaneal tuber	5	Talus
2	Trochlea	6	Tarsal sinus
3	Groove for tendon of M. flexor digitorum profundus	7	Central tarsal bone
		8	Third tarsal bone
4	Calcaneus	9	Fourth tarsal bone

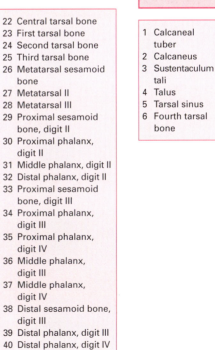

207. Left tarsal bones of pig, plantar view.

1	Calcaneal tuber	7	Central tarsal bone
2	Calcaneus	8	Second tarsal bone
3	Sustentaculum tali	9	First tarsal bone
4	Talus		
5	Tarsal sinus		
6	Fourth tarsal bone		

204. Skeleton of left pelvic limb of pig, lateral view.

205. Skeleton of left pelvic limb of pig, medial view.

Femur
1 Head
2 Greater trochanter
3 Body
4 Trochlea
5 Lateral epicondyle
6 Lateral condyle

Patella
7 Base
8 Apex

Crus
9 Lateral condyle of tibia
10 Tibial tuberosity
11 Head of fibula
12 Interosseous space
13 Body of tibia
14 Body of fibula
15 Lateral malleolus

Pes
16 Calcaneal tuber
17 Talus
18 Calcaneus
19 Central tarsal bone
20 Third tarsal bone
21 Fourth tarsal bone

22 Metatarsal sesamoid bone
23 Metatarsal III
24 Metatarsal IV
25 Metatarsal V
26 Proximal sesamoid bone, digit V
27 Proximal phalanx, digit V
28 Proximal phalanx, digit III
29 Proximal phalanx, digit IV
30 Proximal sesamoid bone, digit IV
31 Middle phalanx, digit V
32 Distal phalanx, digit V
33 Middle phalanx, digit III
34 Middle phalanx, digit IV
35 Distal phalanx, digit III
36 Distal phalanx, digit IV
37 Distal sesamoid bone, digit IV

Femur
1 Head
2 Greater trochanter
3 Trochanteric fossa
4 Neck
5 Lesser trochanter
6 Body
7 Medial supracondyloid tuberosity
8 Trochlea
9 Medial epicondyle
10 Medial condyle

Patella
11 Base
12 Apex

Crus
13 Head of fibula
14 Medial condyle of tibia
15 Tibial tuberosity
16 Body of fibula
17 Body of tibia
18 Medial malleolus

Pes
19 Calcaneal tuber
20 Calcaneus
21 Talus

22 Central tarsal bone
23 First tarsal bone
24 Second tarsal bone
25 Third tarsal bone
26 Metatarsal sesamoid bone
27 Metatarsal II
28 Metatarsal III
29 Proximal sesamoid bone, digit II
30 Proximal phalanx, digit II
31 Middle phalanx, digit II
32 Distal phalanx, digit II
33 Proximal sesamoid bone, digit III
34 Proximal phalanx, digit III
35 Proximal phalanx, digit IV
36 Middle phalanx, digit III
37 Middle phalanx, digit IV
38 Distal sesamoid bone, digit III
39 Distal phalanx, digit III
40 Distal phalanx, digit IV

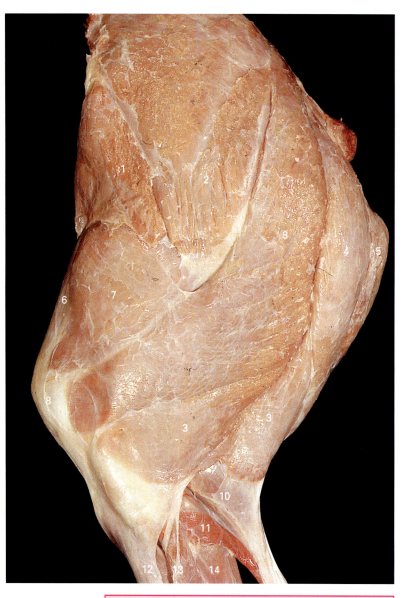

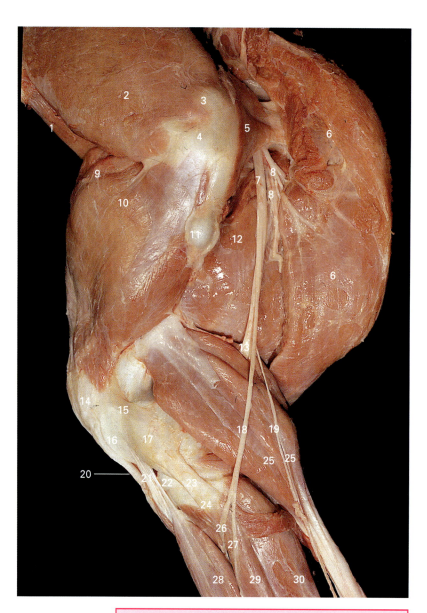

1 M. tensor fascia lata	10 M. gastrocnemius, lateral head
2 M. gluteus superficialis	11 M. soleus
3 M. biceps femoris	12 M. extensor digitorum longus
4 M. semitendinosus	13 M. extensor digitorum lateralis
5 M. semimembranosus	
6 M. rectus femoris	14 M. flexor digitorum profundus
7 M. vastus lateralis	
8 Patella	
9 Lateral condyle of tibia	

1 M. iliacus	19 Caudal cutaneous sural nerve
2 M. gluteus medius	20 Middle patellar ligament
3 Trochanteric bursa	21 Lateral patellar ligament
4 Greater trochanter	22 Lateral meniscus
5 M. piriformis	23 Lateral collateral femorotibial ligament
6 M. semimembranosus	
7 Ischiatic nerve	24 Lateral condyle of tibia
8 Muscular branches of tibial nerve	25 M. gastrocnemius, lateral head
9 M. rectus femoris	26 Deep peroneal (fibular) nerve
10 M. vastus lateralis	
11 Third trochanter	27 Superficial peroneal (fibular) nerve
12 M. adductor	
13 Tibial nerve	28 M. extensor digitorum longus
14 Patella	
15 Lateral femoropatellar ligament	29 M. extensor digitorum lateralis
16 Trochlea of femur	30 M. flexor digitorum profundus
17 Lateral epicondyle of femur	
18 Common peroneal (fibular) nerve	

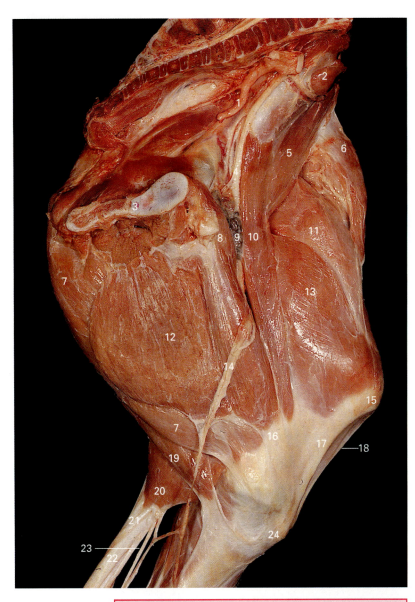

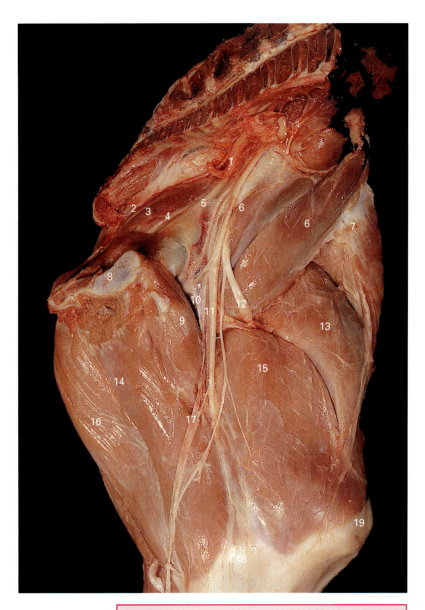

210. Superficial dissection of left pelvis and thigh of foal, medial view. The trunk has been sectioned in a median plane, and the viscera have been removed.

1 Umbilical artery (cut)	15 Patella
2 M. psoas minor	16 Medial epicondyle of femur
3 Pubis	17 Medial patellar ligament
4 Femoral nerve	18 Middle patellar ligament
5 M. iliopsoas	19 M. semitendinosus
6 M. tensor fascia lata	20 M. gastrocnemius, medial head
7 M. semimembranosus	21 Common calcaneal tendon
8 M. pectineus	22 Tendon of M. flexor digitorum superficialis
9 Deep inguinal lymph nodes	23 Tibial nerve
10 M. sartorius	24 Tibial tuberosity
11 M. rectus femoris	
12 M. gracilis	
13 M. vastus medialis	
14 Saphenous vessels and nerve	

211. Deep dissection of left pelvis and thigh of foal, medial view. The trunk has been sectioned in a median plane and the viscera have been removed. The deep inguinal lymph nodes, M. gracilis and M. sartorius have been removed.

1 Umbilical artery (cut)	11 Saphenous nerve
2 Internal iliac artery	12 Femoral nerve
3 M. obturator internus	13 M. rectus femoris
4 Obturator artery	14 M. adductor
5 Obturator nerve	15 M. vastus medialis
6 M. iliopsoas	16 M. semimembranosus
7 M. tensor fascia lata	17 Saphenous vessels
8 Pubis	18 Medial epicondyle of femur
9 M. pectineus	19 Patella
10 Femoral vessels	

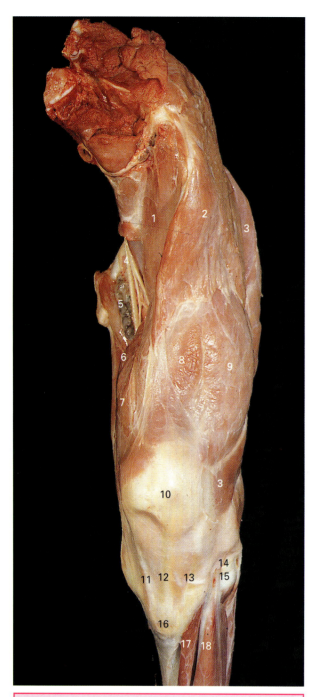

212. **Superficial dissection of left pelvis and thigh of foal, cranial view. The trunk has been sectioned in a median plane and the viscera have been removed. The fascia lata has been removed to expose M. rectus femoris and M. vastus lateralis.**

1 M. iliopsoas	10 Patella
2 M. tensor fascia lata	11 Medial patellar ligament
3 M. biceps femoris	12 Middle patellar ligament
4 Femoral nerve	13 Lateral patellar ligament
5 Deep inguinal lymph	14 Lateral meniscus
nodes	15 Lateral condyle of tibia
6 M. sartorius	16 Tibial tuberosity
7 M. vastus medialis	17 M. tibialis cranialis
8 M. rectus femoris	18 M. extensor digitorum
9 M. vastus lateralis	longus

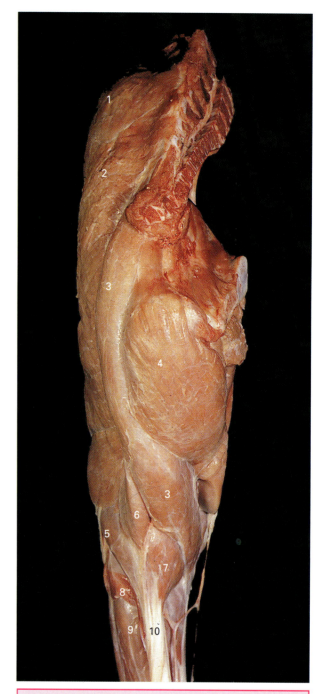

213. **Superficial dissection of left pelvis and thigh of foal, caudal view. The trunk has been sectioned in a median plane, and the viscera have been removed.**

1 M. gluteus superficialis	7 M. gastrocnemius, medial
2 M. biceps femoris	head
3 M. semitendinosus	8 M. soleus
4 M. semimembranosus	9 M. flexor digitorum
5 M. gastrocnemius, lateral	longus
head	10 Common calcaneal
6 M. flexor digitorum	tendon
superficialis	

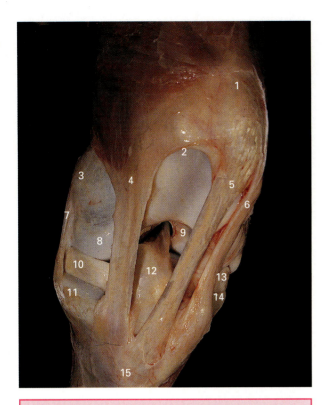

214. Deep dissection of left femorotibial joint of horse, craniomedial view. The joint is partially flexed.

1 Patella	8 Medial condyle of femur
2 Medial trochlear ridge	9 Intercondyloid fossa of
3 Medial epicondyle of	femur
femur	10 Medial meniscus
4 Medial patellar ligament	11 Medial condyle of tibia
5 Middle patellar ligament	12 Cranial cruciate ligament
6 Lateral patellar ligament	13 Lateral meniscus
7 Medial collateral	14 Lateral condyle of tibia
femorotibial ligament	15 Tibial tuberosity

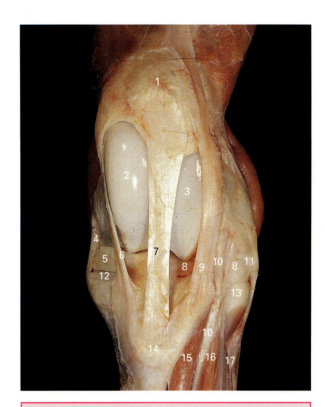

215. Deep dissection of left femorotibial joint of horse, cranial view. The joint is extended with the medial femoral condyle engaged between the middle and medial patellar ligaments.

1 Patella	10 Tendon of M. peroneus
2 Medial trochlear ridge of	(fibularis) tertius
femur	11 Lateral collateral
3 Lateral trochlear ridge of	femorotibial ligament
femur	12 Medial condyle of tibia
4 Medial collateral	13 Lateral condyle of tibia
femorotibial ligament	14 Tibial tuberosity
5 Medial meniscus	15 M. tibialis cranialis
6 Medial patellar ligament	16 M. extensor digitorum
7 Middle patellar ligament	longus
8 Lateral meniscus	17 M. extensor digitorum
9 Lateral patellar ligament	lateralis

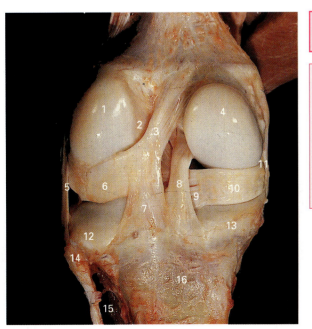

216. Deep dissection of left femorotibial joint of horse, caudal view.

1 Lateral condyle of femur	9 Caudal ligament of
2 Cranial cruciate ligament	medial meniscus
3 Meniscofemoral ligament	10 Medial meniscus
of lateral meniscus	11 Medial collateral
4 Medial condyle of femur	femorotibial ligament
5 Lateral collateral	12 Lateral condyle of tibia
femorotibial ligament	13 Medial condyle of tibia
6 Lateral meniscus	14 Head of fibula
7 Caudal ligament of lateral	15 Interosseous space
meniscus	16 Tibia
8 Caudal cruciate ligament	

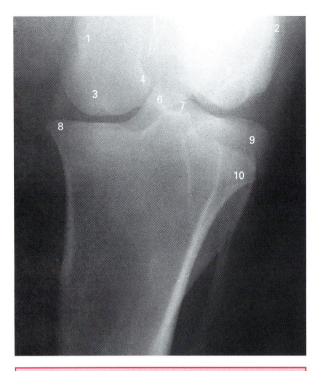

217. Radiograph of left genual joint of horse, craniocaudal projection.

Femur
1 Medial epicondyle
2 Lateral epicondyle
3 Medial condyle
4 Intercondyloid fossa
5 Lateral condyle

Tibia
6 Medial intercondylar tubercle

7 Lateral intercondylar tubercle
8 Medial condyle
9 Lateral condyle

Fibula
10 Head of fibula

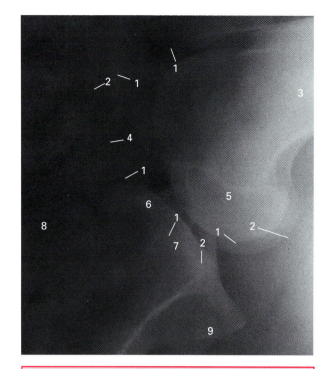

218. Radiograph of left genual joint of horse, lateromedial projection.

Femur
1 Lateral ridge
2 Medial ridge
3 Supracondyloid fossa
4 Trochlear groove
5 Intercondylar fossa
6 Medial intercondylar tubercle

7 Lateral intercondylar tubercle

Tibia
8 Tibial tuberosity
9 Lateral condyle

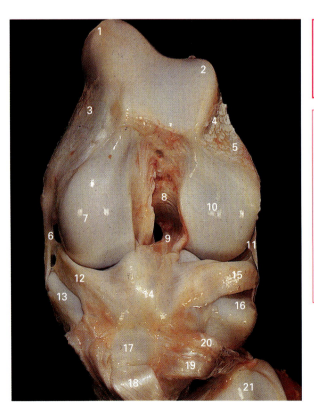

219. Deep dissection of left genual joint of horse, cranial view. The cranial cruciate ligament has been removed, and the patellar ligaments have been cut and reflected distally. The joint is fully flexed to show the distal extremity of the femur.

1 Medial trochlear ridge of femur
2 Lateral trochlear ridge of femur
3 Medial epicondyle
4 Extensor fossa
5 Lateral epicondyle
6 Medial collateral femorotibial ligament
7 Medial condyle of femur
8 Intercondyloid fossa
9 Caudal cruciate ligament
10 Lateral condyle of femur
11 Lateral collateral femorotibial ligament

12 Medial meniscus
13 Medial condyle of tibia
14 Cranial ligaments of menisci
15 Lateral meniscus
16 Lateral condyle of tibia
17 Tibial tuberosity
18 Medial patellar ligament (reflected)
19 Middle patellar ligament (reflected)
20 Lateral patellar ligament (reflected)
21 Articular face of patella

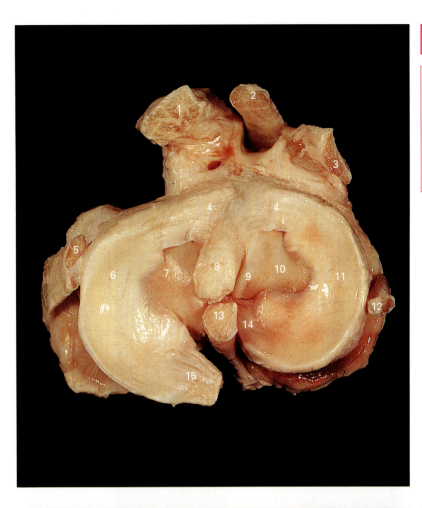

220. Left tibia and menisci of horse, proximal view.

1	Lateral patellar ligament	9	Spine of tibia
2	Middle patellar ligament	10	Medial condyle of tibia
3	Medial patellar ligament	11	Medial meniscus
4	Cranial ligaments of menisci	12	Medial collateral femorotibial ligament
5	Lateral collateral femorotibial ligament	13	Caudal cruciate ligament
6	Lateral meniscus	14	Caudal ligament of medial meniscus
7	Lateral condyle of tibia	15	Meniscofemoral ligament of lateral meniscus
8	Cranial cruciate ligament		

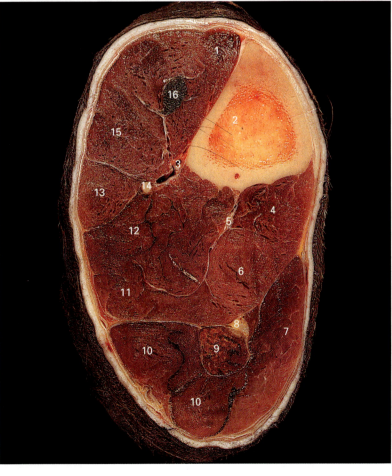

221. Transverse section through left crus of horse at the level of the junction between the proximal and middle third, distal view.

1	M. tibialis cranialis	10	M. gastrocnemius, lateral head
2	Tibia		
3	Cranial tibial vessels	11	M. tibialis caudalis
4	M. popliteus	12	M. flexor digitorum profundus
5	Caudal tibial vessels		
6	M. flexor digitorum longus	13	M. extensor digitorum lateralis
7	M. gastrocnemius, medial head	14	Fibula
8	Tibial nerve	15	M. extensor digitorum longus
9	M. flexor digitorum superficialis	16	M. peroneus (fibularis) tertius

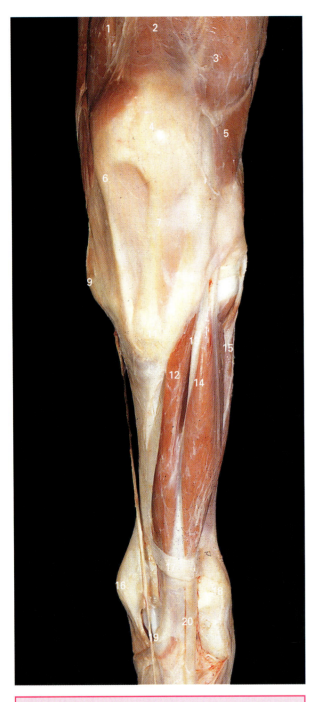

222. Superficial dissection of left crus of horse, cranial view.

1 M. vastus medialis	14 M. extensor digitorum
2 M. rectus femoris	longus
3 M. vastus lateralis	15 M. extensor digitorum
4 Patella	lateralis
5 M. biceps femoris	16 Medial malleolus
6 Medial patellar ligament	17 Proximal extensor
7 Middle patellar ligament	retinaculum of tarsus
8 Lateral patellar ligament	18 Lateral malleolus
9 Medial condyle of tibia	19 Medial tendon of
10 Lateral condyle of tibia	M. tibialis cranialis
11 Tibial tuberosity	(cunean tendon)
12 M. tibialis cranialis	20 Tendon of M. extensor
13 Tendon of M. peroneus	digitorum longus
(fibularis) tertius	

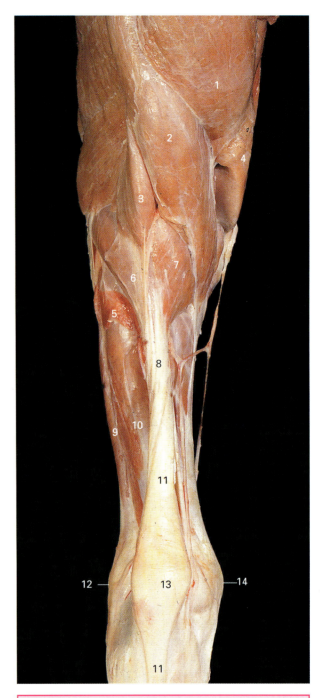

223. Superficial dissection of left crus of horse, caudal view.

1 M. semimembranosus	9 M. extensor digitorum
2 M. semitendinosus	lateralis
3 M. biceps femoris	10 M. flexor digitorum
4 M. gracilis	profundus
5 M. soleus	11 Tendon of M. flexor
6 M. gastrocnemius, lateral	digitorum superficialis
head	12 Lateral malleolus
7 M. gastrocnemius, medial	13 Calcaneal tuber
head	14 Medial malleolus
8 Common calcaneal tendon	

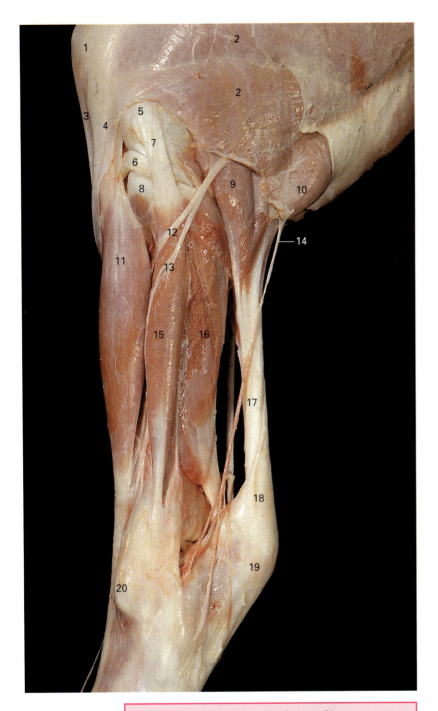

224. Superficial dissection of left crus of horse, lateral view.

1 Patella	13 Superficial peroneal (fibular) nerve
2 M. biceps femoris	
3 Middle patellar ligament	14 Caudal cutaneous sural nerve
4 Lateral patellar ligament	
5 Lateral epicondyle of femur	15 M. extensor digitorum lateralis
6 Lateral meniscus	16 M. flexor digitorum profundus
7 Lateral collateral femorotibial ligament	17 Common calcanean tendon
8 Lateral condyle of tibia	18 Tendon of M. flexor digitorum superficialis
9 M. gastrocnemius, lateral head	
10 M. semitendinosus	19 Calcaneal tuber
11 M. extensor digitorum longus	20 Lateral malleolus
12 Deep peroneal (fibular) nerve	

225. Superficial dissection of left crus of horse, medial view.

1 M. semimembranosus	6 Tendon of M. flexor digitorum superficialis
2 M. semitendinosus	
3 M. gastrocnemius, medial head	7 Tibial nerve
4 Common calcanean tendon	8 Saphenous artery
5 Medial saphenous vein, cranial branch	9 Medial saphenous vein, caudal branch
	10 Calcaneal tuber
	11 Medial malleolus

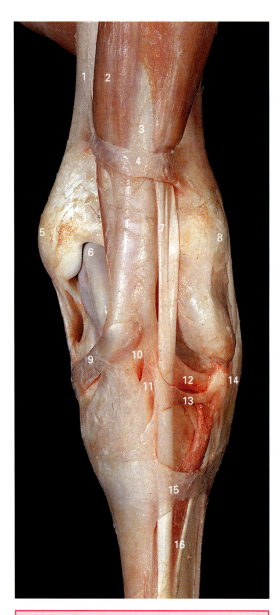

226. Superficial dissection of left tarsus of horse, dorsal view.

1 Tibia	10 Dorsal tendon of
2 M. tibialis cranialis	M. peroneus
3 Tendon of M. peroneus	(fibularis) tertius
(fibularis) tertius	11 Dorsal tendon of
4 Proximal extensor	M. tibialis cranialis
retinaculum	12 Lateral tendon of
5 Medial malleolus	M. peroneus
6 Trochlea of talus	(fibularis) tertius
7 Tendon of M. extensor	13 Middle extensor
digitorum longus	retinaculum
8 Lateral malleolus	14 Long lateral collateral
9 Medial tendon of M.	tarsal ligament
tibialis cranialis	15 Distal extensor
(cunean tendon)	retinaculum
	16 Tendon of M. extensor
	digitorum lateralis

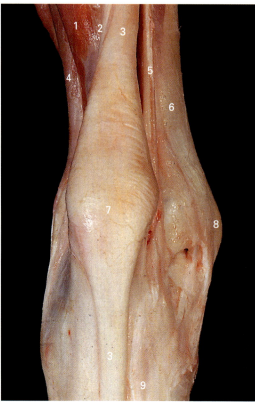

227. Superficial dissection of left tarsus of horse, plantar view.

1 M. flexor digitorum	5 M. flexor digitorum
profundus, superficial	profundus, medial head
head	6 Tibia
2 Tendon of M.	7 Calcaneal tuber
gastrocnemius	8 Medial malleolus
3 Tendon of M. flexor	9 Tendon of M. flexor
digitorum superficialis	digitorum profundus
4 M. extensor digitorum	
lateralis	

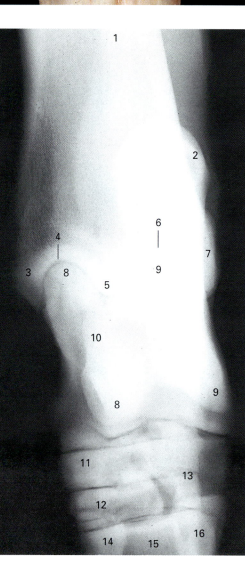

228. Radiograph of left tarsus of horse, dorsoplantar projection.

1 Tibia	11 Central tarsal bone
2 Calcaneus	12 Third tarsal bone
3 Medial malleolus	13 Fourth tarsal bone
4 Medial groove	14 Metatarsal II (medial
5 Sagittal ridge	splint bone)
6 Lateral groove	15 Metatarsal III (cannon
7 Lateral malleolus	bone)
8 Medial ridge of talus	16 Metatarsal IV (lateral
9 Lateral ridge of talus	splint bone)
10 Sustentaculum tali	

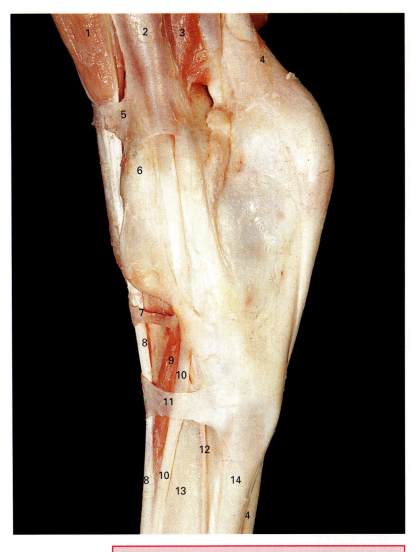

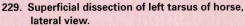

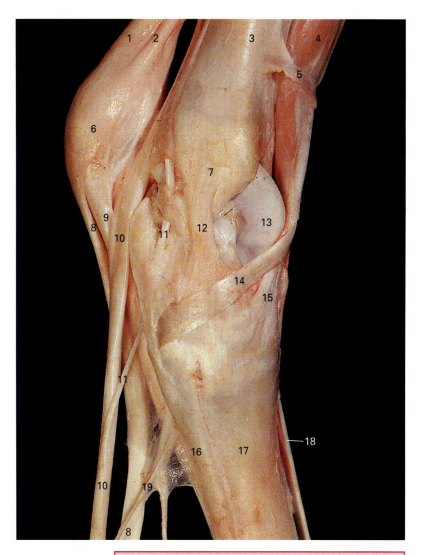

229. Superficial dissection of left tarsus of horse, lateral view.

1 M. tibialis cranialis	9 M. extensor digitorum brevis
2 M. extensor digitorum lateralis	10 Tendon of M. extensor digitorum lateralis
3 M. flexor digitorum profundus	11 Distal extensor retinaculum
4 Tendon of M. flexor digitorum superficialis	12 Dorsal metatarsal artery III
5 Proximal extensor retinaculum	13 Metatarsal III (cannon bone)
6 Lateral malleolus	14 Metatarsal IV (lateral splint bone)
7 Middle extensor retinaculum	
8 Tendon of M. extensor digitorum longus	

230. Superficial dissection of left tarsus of horse, medial view. Tendons of M. flexor digitorum profundus and M. flexor digitorum superficialis have been retracted in a plantar direction in the metatarsal region.

1 Tendon of M. flexor digitorum superficialis	13 Trochlea of talus
2 Tendon of M. gastrocnemius	14 Medial tendon of M. tibialis cranialis (cunean tendon)
3 Tibia	15 Dorsal tendon of M. peroneus (fibularis) longus
4 M. tibialis cranialis	
5 Proximal extensor retinaculum	16 Metatarsal II (medial splint bone)
6 Calcaneal tuber	17 Metatarsal III (cannon bone)
7 Medial malleolus	
8 Tendon of M. flexor digitorum superficialis	18 Tendon of M. extensor digitorum longus
9 Plantar ligament	19 Accessory ligament of M. flexor digitorum profundus (distal check ligament)
10 Tendon of M. flexor digitorum profundus	
11 Tendon of M. flexor digitorum longus	
12 Medial collateral tarsal ligament	

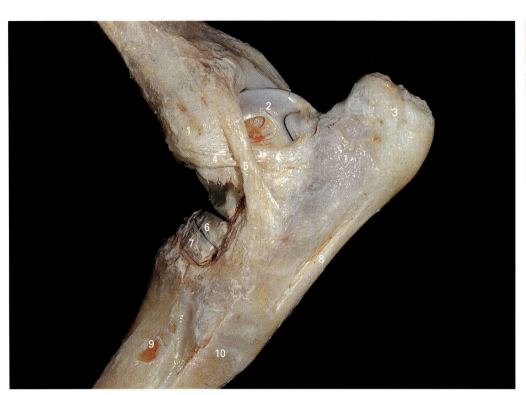

231. Deep dissection of left tarsus of horse, flexed lateral view.

1 Lateral malleolus
2 Lateral ridge of trochlea of talus
3 Calcaneal tuber
4 Short lateral collateral tarsal ligament
5 Long lateral collateral tarsal ligament
6 Central tarsal bone
7 Third tarsal bone
8 Long plantar ligament
9 Metatarsal III (cannon bone)
10 Metatarsal IV (lateral splint bone)

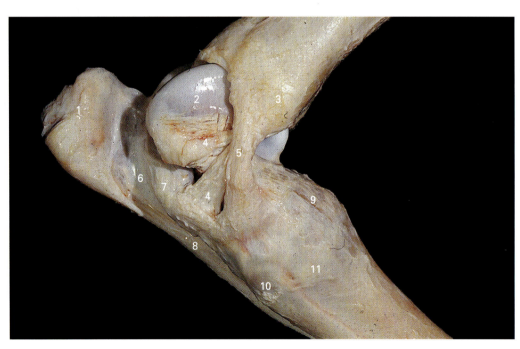

232. Deep dissection of left tarsus of horse, medial view of flexed joint.

1 Calcaneal tuber
2 Medial ridge of trochlea of talus
3 Medial malleolus
4 Short medial collateral tarsal ligament
5 Long medial collateral tarsal ligament
6 Groove for tendon of M. flexor digitorum profundus
7 Sustentaculum tali
8 Long plantar ligament
9 Dorsal tarsal ligament
10 Metatarsal II (medial splint bone)
11 Metatarsal III (cannon bone)

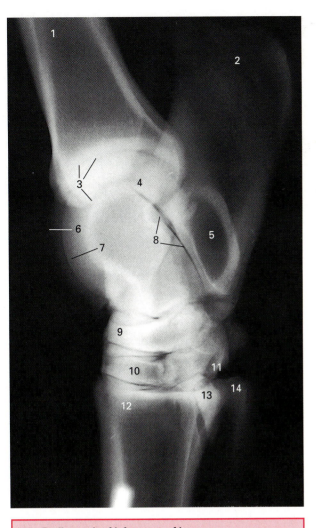

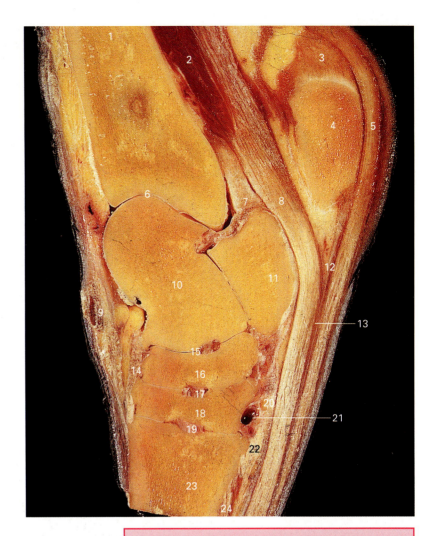

233. Radiograph of left tarsus of horse, lateromedial projection.

234. Sagittal section through left tarsus of horse.

1 Tibia	9 Central tarsal bone
2 Calcaneus	10 Third tarsal bone
3 Tarsocrural joint	11 First and second tarsal bone (fused)
4 Coracoid process of calcaneus	12 Metatarsal III (cannon bone)
5 Sustentaculum tali	13 Metatarsal II (medial splint bone)
6 Medial ridge of trochlea of talus	14 Metatarsal IV (lateral splint bone)
7 Lateral ridge of trochlea of talus	
8 Talocalcaneal joint	

1 Tibia	14 Fibrous joint capsule
2 M. flexor digitorum profundus	15 Proximal intertarsal joint
3 Tendon of M. gastrocnemius	16 Central tarsal bone
4 Calcaneal tuber	17 Distal intertarsal joint
5 Tendon of M. flexor digitorum superficialis	18 Third tarsal bone
6 Tarsocrural joint	19 Tarsometatarsal joint
7 Thick part of joint capsule	20 Joint capsule (tarsometatarsal ligament)
8 Tendon of M. flexor digitorum profundus	21 Proximal perforating tarsal vein
9 Medial tendon of M. tibialis cranialis (cunean tendon)	22 Accessory ligament of M. flexor digitorum profundus (distal check ligament)
10 Talus	23 Metatarsal III (cannon bone)
11 Sustentaculum tali	24 M. interosseus medius (suspensory ligament)
12 Long plantar ligament	
13 Flexor retinaculum	

6 Viscera of the Thorax, Abdomen, and Pelvis

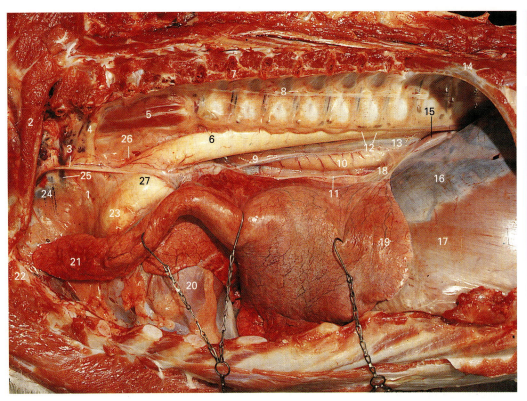

235. Left view of the thorax of a horse. Ribs 2–12 and the associated soft tissues have been removed to expose the thoracic viscera. The left lung has been reflected ventrally.

1 Thymus
2 Rib 1
3 Vagosympathetic trunk
4 Costocervical trunk
5 M. longus colli
6 Aorta
7 Cut dorsal end of rib 7
8 Sympathetic trunk
9 Dorsal trunk of the vagus nerve
10 Oesophagus
11 Ventral trunk of the vagus nerve
12 Aortic lymph nodes
13 Caudal mediastinum
14 Rib 13
15 Left crus of the diaphragm
16 Tendinous centre of the diaphragm
17 Costal part of the diaphragm
18 Ligament of the lung
19 Caudal lobe of the left lung
20 Heart lying in the cardiac notch of the lung and surrounded by the pericardium
21 Reflected cranial lobe of the lung
22 Cut costal cartilage of rib 2
23 Pulmonary trunk
24 Cranial vena cava
25 Costocervical trunk
26 Thoracic duct
27 Arterial ligament

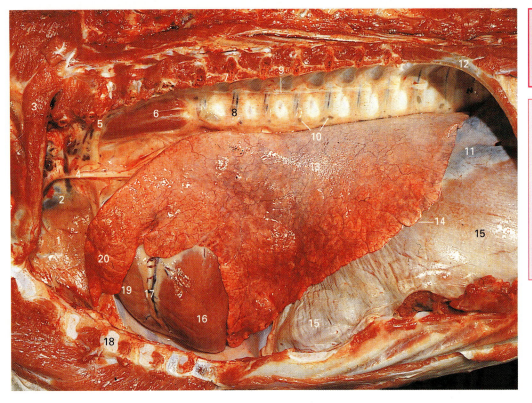

236. Left view of the thorax of a horse. Ribs 2–12 and the associated soft tissues have been removed to expose the thoracic viscera. The left side of the pericardial sac has been removed to partially expose the heart.

1 Thymus
2 Cranial vena cava
3 Rib 1
4 Vagosympathetic trunk
5 Costocervical trunk
6 M. longus colli
7 Cut dorsal end of rib 7
8 Intercostal vessels lying caudal to rib 7
9 Sympathetic trunk
10 Aortic lymph nodes
11 Tendinous centre of the diaphragm
12 Rib 13
13 Caudal lobe of the left lung
14 Basal border of the left lung
15 Costal part of the diaphragm
16 Left ventricle
17 Paraconal interventricular groove
18 Cut cartilage of rib 4
19 Right ventricle
20 Cranial lobe of the left lung

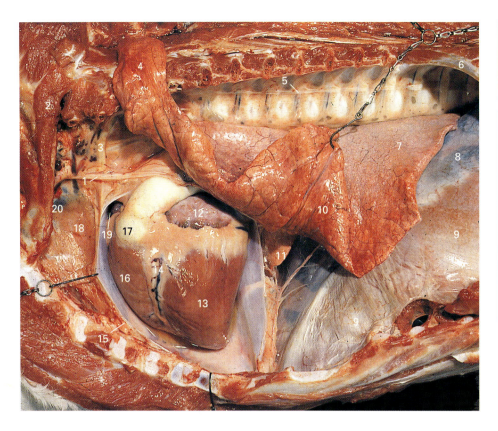

237. Left view of the thorax of a horse. Ribs 2–12 and the associated soft tissues have been removed to expose the thoracic viscera. The left side of the pericardial sac has been removed and the lung has be reflected dorsally.

1 Vagosympathetic trunk
2 Rib 1
3 Costocervical trunk
4 Reflected cranial lobe of the left lung
5 Sympathetic trunk
6 Rib 13
7 Caudal lobe of the left lung
8 Tendinous centre of the diaphragm
9 Costal part of the diaphragm
10 Mediastinal surface of the reflected caudal lobe of the left lung
11 Accessory lobe of the right lung seen through the caudal mediastinum
12 Left auricle
13 Left ventricle
14 Paraconal interventricular groove
15 Cut edge of the pericardial sac
16 Right ventricle
17 Beginning of the pulmonary trunk
18 Thymus
19 Left extremity of the right auricle
20 Cranial vena cava

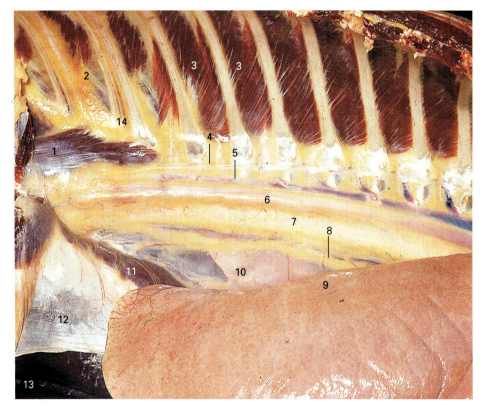

238. The caudodorsal part of the thoracic cavity of a horse seen from the right side. The caudal lobe of the lung has relaxed revealing the structures of the caudal mediastinum.

1 Cranial end of the M. iliopsoas
2 M. intercostalis externus, visible owing to the absence of M. intercostalis internus muscles at this location
3 M. intercostalis internus
4 Sympathetic trunk
5 Azygos vein
6 Thoracic duct
7 Aorta
8 Lymphatics within the caudal mediastinum
9 Dorsal border of the caudal lobe of the right lung
10 Left lung visible through the caudal mediastinum
11 Right crus of the diaphragm
12 Tendinous centre of the diaphragm
13 Liver, exposed by excision of part of the diaphragm
14 Intercostal vessels lying caudal to rib 16

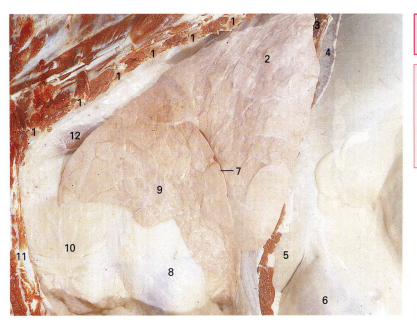

239. Left lateral view of the thorax of a one-year-old bull with ribs 2–13 removed.

1 The cut ends of ribs 2–8
2 Caudal lobe of the left lung
3 Costal part of the diaphragm
4 Spleen
5 Reticulum
6 Abomasum
7 Fissure between cranial and caudal lobes
8 Pericardium
9 Cranial lobe of the left lung
10 Cranial mediastinum
11 Rib 1
12 M. longus colli

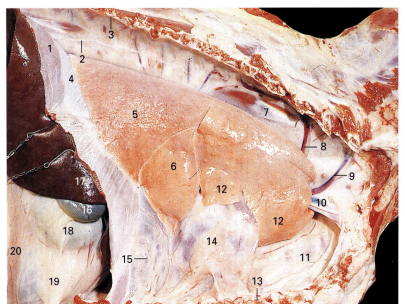

240. Right view of the thorax of the sheep. The thoracic wall has been completely removed.

1 Peripheral muscle of the diaphragm
2 Sympathetic trunk
3 Cut proximal end of rib 10
4 Tendinous centre of the diaphragm
5 Caudal lobe of the right lung
6 Middle lobe of the right lung
7 M. longus colli
8 Right azygos vein
9 Costocervical trunk
10 Cranial vena cava
11 Cranial mediastinum lying against the medial aspect of the left thoracic wall
12 Cranial and caudal divisions of the cranial lobe of the right lung
13 Cut distal end of the cartilage of rib 4
14 Pericardium
15 Caval fold of the pleura
16 Gall bladder
17 Right lobe of the liver
18 Omasum covered by the lesser omentum
19 Reticulum covered by the lesser omentum
20 Duodenum

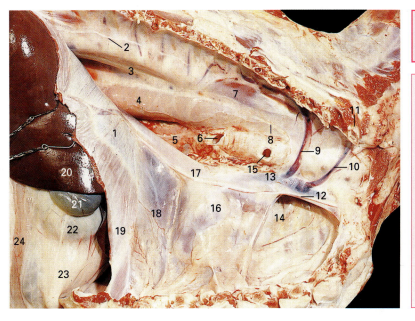

241. Right view of the thorax of the sheep. The thoracic wall and the right lung have been completely removed.

1 Tendinous centre of the diaphragm
2 Sympathetic trunk
3 Thoracic duct
4 Oesophagus
5 Left lung visible through the caudal mediastinum
6 Cut right principal bronchus
7 M. longus colli
8 Dorsal trunk of vagus nerve
9 Right azygos vein
10 Costocervical trunk
11 Cut proximal end of rib 1
12 Right phrenic nerve
13 Cranial vena cava
14 Cranial mediastinum lying against the medial aspect of the left thoracic wall
15 Cut tracheal bronchus supplying the cranial lobe of the right lung
16 Pericardium
17 Caudal vena cava accompanied by the right phrenic nerve
18 Caval fold of the pleura
19 Costal part of the diaphragm
20 Right lobe of the liver
21 Gall bladder
22 Omasum covered by the lesser omentum
23 Reticulum covered by the lesser omentum
24 Duodenum

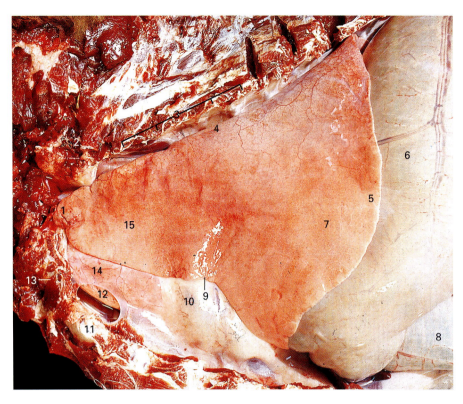

242. Left view of the thoracic region of a llama with the thoracic wall removed. The cut costal part of the diaphragm has slipped from view between the lung and the first compartment of the stomach.

1 Apex of the lung	10 Lateral surface of the pericardium
2 Point of attachment of the head of rib 1	11 Sternal attachment of rib 2
3 Ribs 2–5 in section	12 Cranial lobe of the right lung seen through an opening in the cranial mediastinum
4 Dorsal border of the lung	
5 Basal border of the lung	
6 First compartment of the stomach	13 Cut ventral end of rib 1
7 Caudal lobe of the left lung	14 Cranial mediastinum
8 Third compartment of the stomach	15 Cranial lobe of the left lung
9 Cardiac notch	

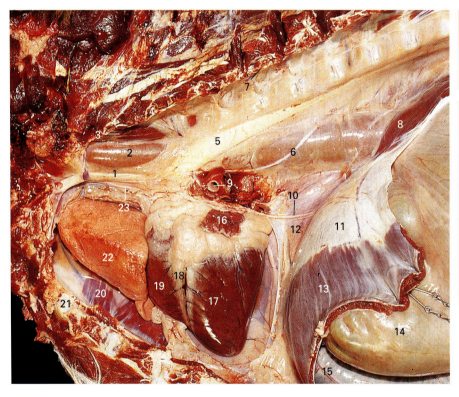

243. Left view of the thorax of a llama with the left lung and thoracic wall removed. The left side of the pericardium and the membranous part of the cranial mediastinum have been removed, revealing the heart and part of the right lung.

1 Brachiocephalic trunk	14 First compartment of the stomach
2 Oesophagus	15 Third compartment of the stomach
3 M. longus colli	
4 Ribs 2–4 in section	16 Left auricle
5 Aorta	17 Left ventricle
6 Dorsal trunk of the vagus nerve	18 Paraconal interventricular groove
7 Sympathetic trunk	19 Right ventricle
8 Left crus of the diaphragm	20 Part of M. transversus thoracis
9 Left bronchus in section	
10 Left phrenic nerve	21 Sternal attachment of rib 2
11 Tendinous centre of the diaphragm	22 Cranial lobe of the right lung
12 Caudal mediastinum	
13 Costal part of the diaphragm	23 Vagosympathetic trunk

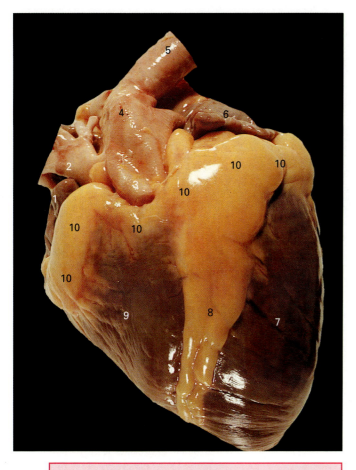

---

244. Left view of the equine heart.

1 Right auricle	7 Left ventricle
2 Brachiocephalic trunk	8 Paraconal interventricular
3 Pulmonary trunk	groove
4 Arterial ligament	9 Right ventricle
5 Aorta	10 Coronary groove
6 Left auricle	

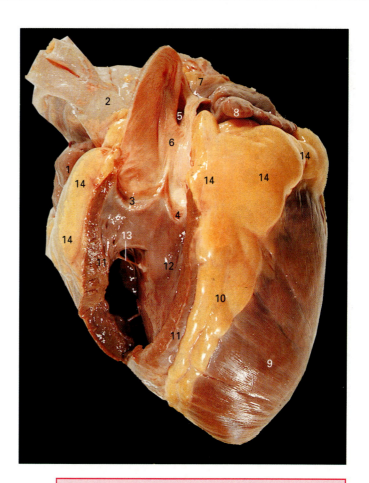

**245. Left view of the equine heart with part of the wall
of the right ventricle removed.**

1 Right auricle	6 Pulmonary trunk
2 Brachiocephalic trunk	7 Part of the left atrium
3 Intermediate cusp of the	8 Left auricle
pulmonary valve	9 Left ventricle
4 Right cusp of the	10 Paraconal interventricular
pulmonary valve	groove
5 Depression marking the	11 Wall of the right ventricle
attachment of the arterial	12 Interventricular septum
ligament to the outside of	13 Septomarginal band
the vessel	14 Coronary groove

**246. The equine heart sectioned transversely through
the left atrioventricular valve. The specimen is
viewed from behind.**

1 Cut wall of the left	6 Part of the interatrial
ventricle	septum
2 Fat filling the coronary	7 Septal cusp of the left
groove	atrioventricular valve
3 Cut wall of the left atrium	8 Arrow pointing towards
4 Interior of the left atrium	the aortic valve
5 Interior of the left auricle	9 Papillary muscle
showing pectinate muscles	10 Tendinous cords

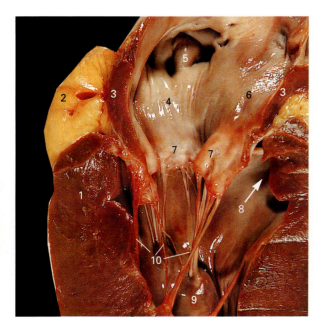

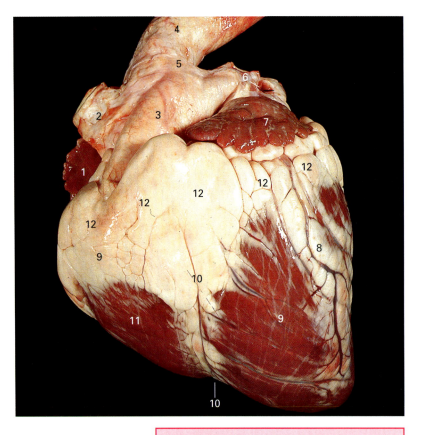
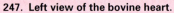

247. Left view of the bovine heart.

1 Right auricle	8 Intermediate groove
2 Brachiocephalic trunk	9 Left ventricle
3 Pulmonary trunk	10 Paraconal
4 Aorta	interventricular
5 Arterial ligament	groove
6 One of many	11 Right ventricle
pulmonary veins	12 Coronary groove
entering the left atrium	
7 Left auricle	

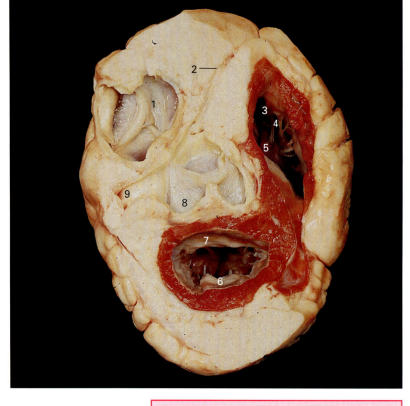

248. Dorsal view of the base of the bovine heart. The atria and great vessels have been removed. The cranial aspect is towards the top of the page.

1 Pulmonary valve	6 Left atrioventricular
2 Right coronary artery	valve, parietal cusp
3 Right atrioventricular	7 Left atrioventricular
valve	valve, septal cusp
4 Tendinous cords	8 Aortic valve
5 Papillary muscle	9 Left coronary artery

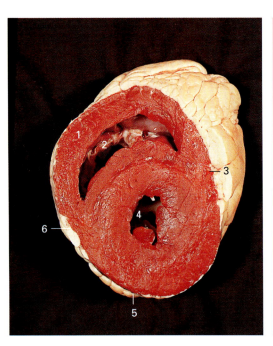

249. Dorsal section through ventricles of bovine heart at a point midway between the apex and the coronary groove. The cranial aspect is towards the top of the page. Ventral view.

1 Parietal wall of the right ventricle
2 Lumen of the right ventricle
3 Paraconal interventricular groove
4 Lumen of the left ventricle
5 Intermediate groove
6 Subsinual interventricular groove

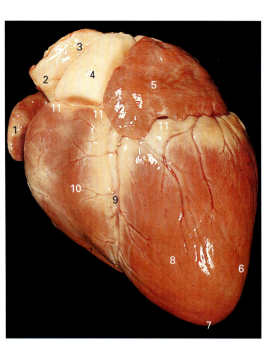

250. Left view of a porcine heart.

1 Right auricle
2 Brachiocephalic trunk
3 Aorta
4 Pulmonary trunk
5 Left auricle
6 Caudal border of the left ventricle
7 Apex of the left ventricle
8 Left ventricle
9 Paraconal interventricular groove
10 Right ventricle
11 Coronary groove

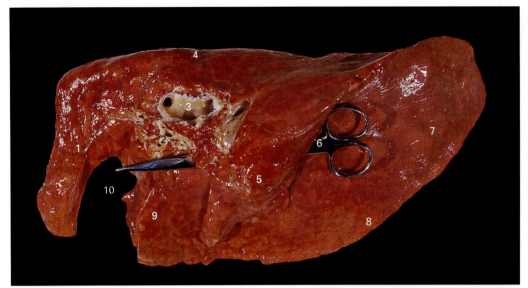

251. Medial view of the right lung of the horse.

1 Cranial lobe
2 Pulmonary arteries
3 Right principal bronchus with its medial wall removed
4 Dorsal border
5 Accessory lobe

6 Scissors indicating the course followed by the caudal vena cava
7 Diaphragmatic surface of the caudal lobe
8 Basal border
9 Middle lobe
10 Cardiac notch

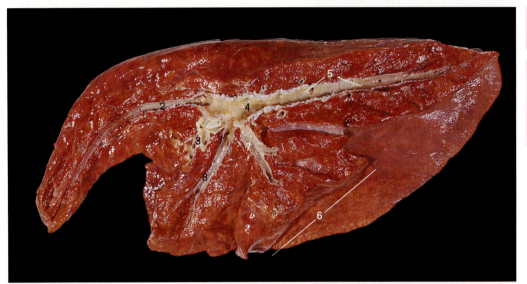

252. Medial view of the right lung of the horse dissected to show the lobar bronchi.

1 Cranial lobe
2 Cranial lobar bronchus
3 Pulmonary arteries
4 Caudal lobar bronchus
5 Segmental bronchi leaving the caudal lobar bronchus

6 Accessory lobe
7 Accessory lobar bronchus
8 Middle lobar bronchus

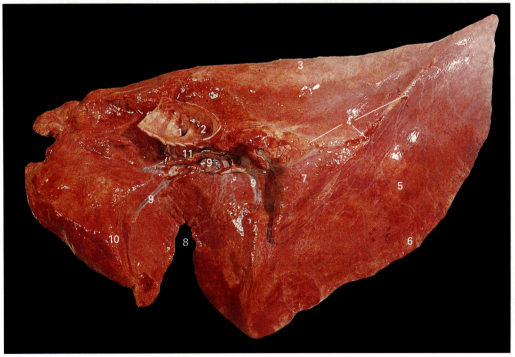

253. Medial view of the right lung of a llama. A little of the right terminal part of the trachea has been left in place. Owing to the absence of interlobar fissures, the middle lobe cannot be precisely defined from the exterior and it has been left unlabelled.

1 Right cranial lobar bronchus
2 Origin of the middle, caudal and accessory lobar bronchi
3 Dorsal border of the lung
4 Cut attachment of the ligament of the lung

5 Diaphragmatic surface of the caudal lobe
6 Basal border of the lung
7 Accessory lobe
8 Cardiac notch
9 Pulmonary veins
10 Cranial lobe
11 Point of entry of the pulmonary artery

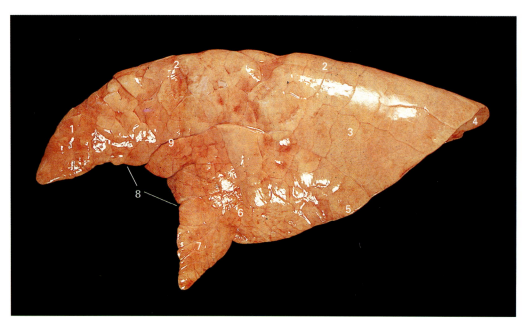

254. Lateral view of the left lung of a pig.

1 Cranial division of the
   cranial lobe
2 Dorsal border
3 Costal surface of the
   caudal lobe
4 Diaphragmatic surface of
   the caudal lobe
5 Basal border of the lung

6 Fissure dividing the
   cranial and caudal lobes
7 Caudal division of the
   cranial lobe
8 Cardiac notch
9 Fissure dividing the
   cranial and caudal
   divisions of the cranial
   lobe

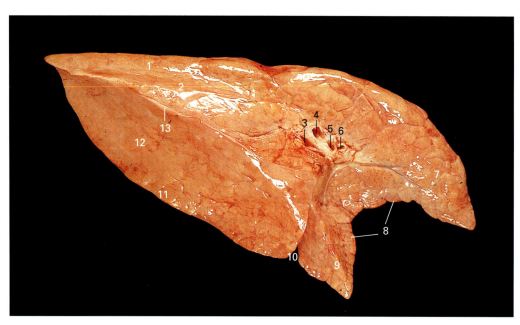

255. Medial view of the left lung of a pig.

1 Dorsal border
2 Aortic impression
3 Pulmonary veins
4 Caudal lobar bronchus
5 Cranial lobar bronchus
6 Pulmonary artery
7 Cranial division of the
   cranial lobe
8 Cardiac notch

9 Caudal division of the
   cranial lobe
10 Fissure dividing the
   cranial and caudal lobes
11 Basal border
12 Diaphragmatic surface of
   the caudal lobe
13 Line of attachment of the
   ligament of the lung

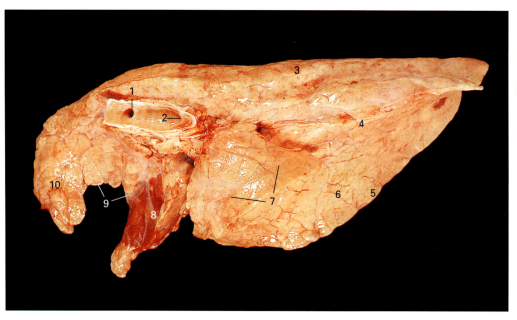

**256. Medial view of the right lung of a pig. The right
lateral wall of the caudal end of the trachea has
been left in place.**

1 Tracheal bronchus
2 Position of the middle,
   caudal and accessory lobar
   bronchi
3 Dorsal border
4 Line of attachment of the
   ligament of the lung

5 Basal border
6 Diaphragmatic surface of
   the caudal lobe
7 Accessory lobe
8 Middle lobe
9 Cardiac notch
10 Cranial lobe

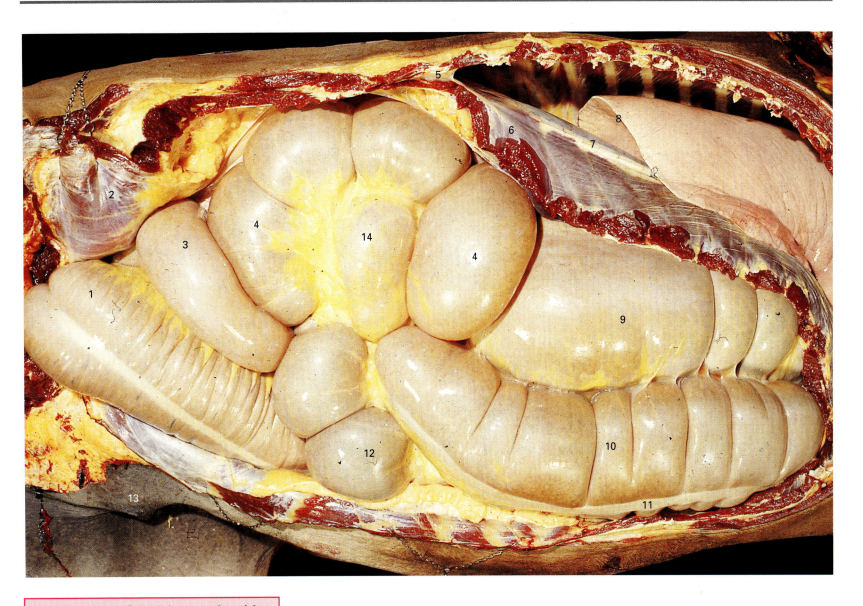

257. The contents of the abdomen and caudal thorax of a large horse seen from the right side after removal of the body wall. The viscera were photographed as they were when the abdomen was opened. The colon and caecum are somewhat distended by enteric gas.

1 Left ventral part of the ascending colon
2 M. abdominis obliquus internus, reflected and seen from the medial aspect through the peritoneum
3 Left dorsal part of the ascending colon
4 Base of the caecum
5 Cut dorsal end of rib 18
6 Costal part of the diaphragm
7 Tendinous centre of the diaphragm
8 Basal border of the right lung
9 Right dorsal part of the ascending colon
10 Right ventral part of the ascending colon
11 Lateral free muscular band of the ascending colon
12 Body of the caecum, the apex lies behind the right ventral part of the colon
13 Mammary gland
14 Beginning of the right ventral part of the ascending colon

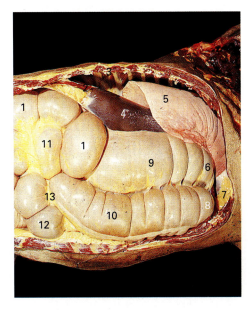

258. The contents of the caudal thorax and cranial abdomen of a large horse seen from the right side after removal of the body wall. The right side of the diaphragm has been removed to reveal the liver and parts of the colon.

1 Base of the caecum
2 Right crus of diaphragm seen in paramedian section
3 Cut dorsal end of rib 16
4 Right lateral lobe of liver
5 Caudal lobe of the right lung
6 Diaphragmatic flexure of the ascending colon
7 Heart enclosed in the pericardium
8 Sternal flexure of the ascending colon
9 Right dorsal part of the ascending colon
10 Right ventral part of the ascending colon
11 Beginning of the right ventral part of the ascending colon
12 Body of the caecum; the apex lies behind the right ventral part of the colon
13 Caecocolic fold

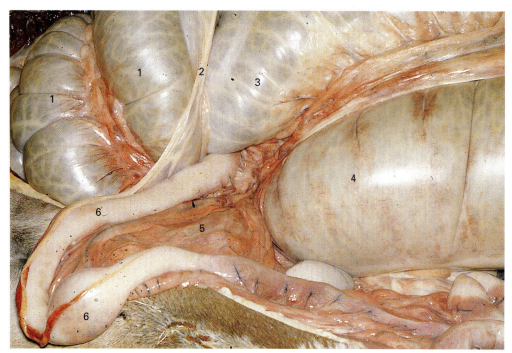

259. Right view of the ileum of the horse.
Both the caecum and the ascending colon have been lifted out of the abdomen and reflected dorsally but none of their attachments have been cut.

1 Caecum
2 Ileocaecal fold
3 Right ventral part of the ascending colon
4 Right dorsal part of the ascending colon at its junction with the transverse colon
5 Mesentery
6 Ileum

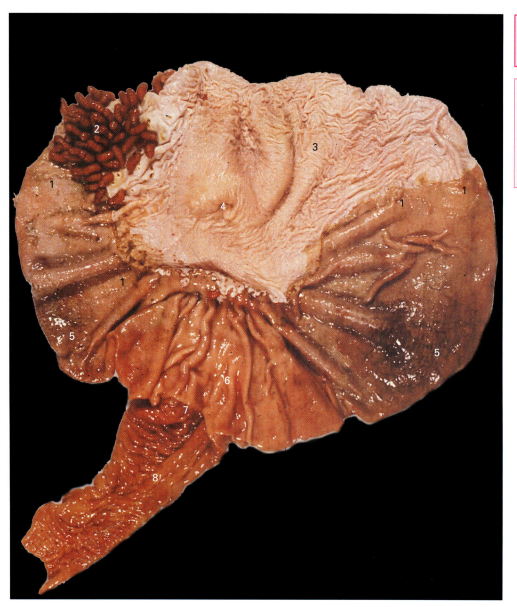

260. The stomach and part of the duodenum of the horse opened to show the mucosa. The stomach was opened along the greater curvature.

1 Cardiac gland area
2 Gastrophilus larvae attached to part of the cardiac gland area
3 Nonglandular part of the stomach lined by keratinized squamous epithelium
4 Cardia
5 Proper gastric gland area
6 Pyloric gland area
7 Pylorus
8 Duodenal mucosa

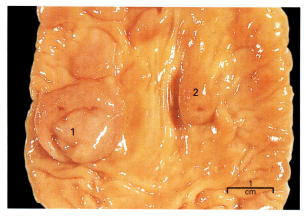

261. Detail of the duodenum of the horse showing the duodenal papillae.

1 Major duodenal papilla
2 Minor duodenal papilla

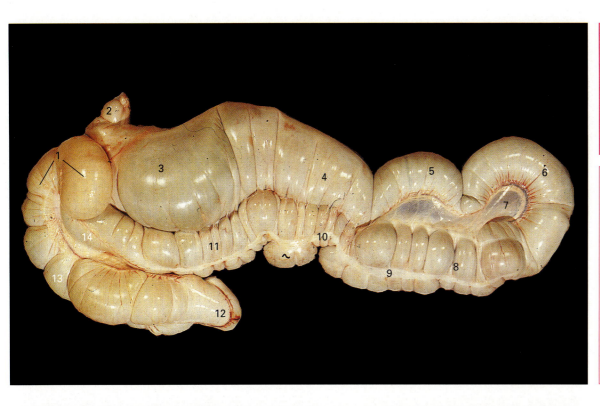

262. The caecum and ascending colon of a four-month-old foal. The organs have been removed from the abdomen and the sternal and diaphragmatic flexures have been straightened. The surfaces shown are normally lateral; thus the part on the left of the photograph lies against the right flank, and that on the right lies against the left flank.

1 Base of the caecum
2 Beginning of the descending colon
3 Confluence of the ascending colon and the transverse colon
4 Diaphragmatic flexure
5 Left dorsal part of the ascending colon
6 Pelvic flexure
7 Mesocolon
8 Left ventral part of the ascending colon
9 Lateral free muscular band
10 Sternal flexure
11 Right ventral part of the ascending colon
12 Apex of the caecum
13 Body of the caecum
14 Beginning of the right ventral part of the ascending colon

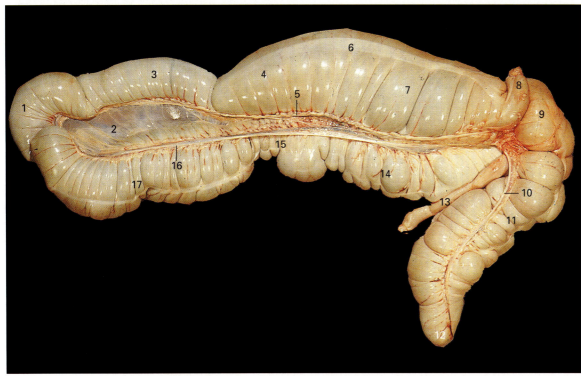

263. The caecum and ascending colon of a four-month-old foal. The organs have been removed from the abdomen and the sternal and diaphragmatic flexures have been straightened. The surfaces shown normally face medially and are related to each other or to loops of the small intestine or descending colon.

1 Pelvic flexure
2 Mesocolon
3 Left dorsal part of the ascending colon
4 Diaphragmatic flexure
5 Right colic artery
6 Medial free muscular band
7 Right dorsal part of the ascending colon close to the junction with the transverse colon
8 Beginning of the descending colon
9 Base of the caecum
10 Medial caecal artery
11 Body of the caecum
12 Apex of the caecum
13 Ileum
14 Right ventral part of the ascending colon
15 Sternal flexure
16 Colic branch of the ileocolic artery
17 Left ventral part of the ascending colon

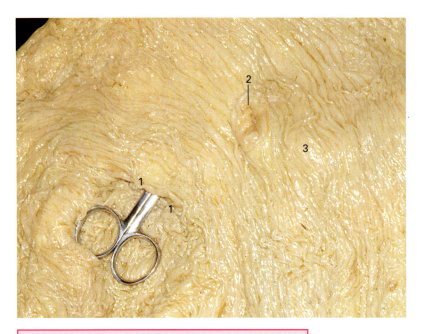

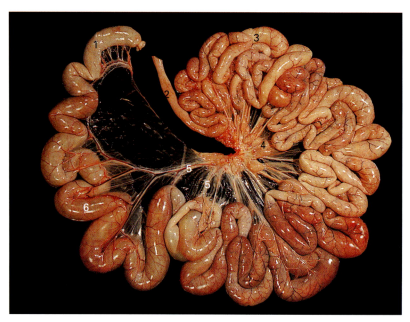

264. The base of the caecum of the horse opened from above to show the mucosa and its continuity with the ileum and right ventral colon.

1 The scissors lie in the caecocolic orifice which is a relatively large, slit-like opening
2 Ileocaecal orifice on a low projection
3 Artefactual ridge caused by the underlying ileum

265. The small intestine of a four-month-old foal removed from the abdomen and spread out as much as the mesentery will allow.

1 Terminal part of the ileum
2 Terminal part of the ascending duodenum
3 Beginning of the jejunum
4 Mesenteric lymph nodes
5 Jejunal blood vessels
6 Terminal part of the jejunum

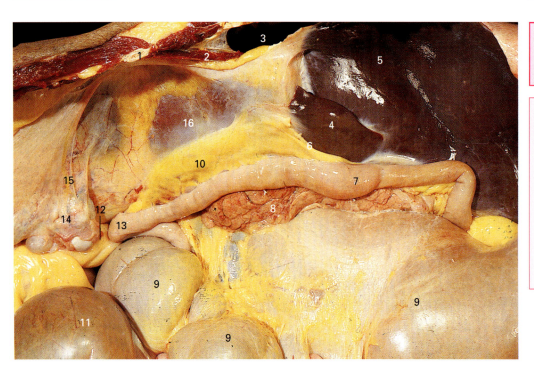

266. Ventrolateral view of the right dorsal part of the abdomen of a mare. The right lateral lobe of the liver has been reflected dorsally and the base of the caecum has been compressed and drawn a little ventrally.

1 Cut dorsal end of rib 18
2 Right crus of the diaphragm in paramedian section
3 Extreme caudodorsal part of the pleural cavity
4 Caudate lobe of the liver
5 Visceral surface of the right lateral lobe of the liver
6 Position of the omental (epiploic) foramen
7 Duodenum
8 Right lobe of the pancreas
9 Base of the caecum
10 Mesoduodenum
11 Loop of the left dorsal part of the ascending colon
12 Uterine tube (oviduct)
13 Duodenal flexure
14 Ovary
15 Suspensory ligament of the ovary
16 Ventral surface of the right kidney

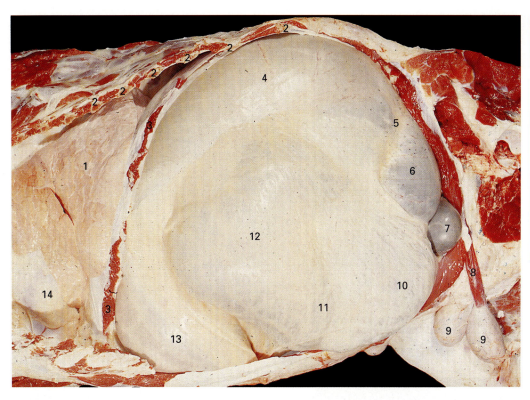

1 Caudal lobe of the left lung
2 The cut ends of ribs 8–13
3 The costal part of the diaphragm
4 Dorsal sac of the rumen
5 Left dorsal coronary groove
6 Caudodorsal blind sac
7 Apex of the caecum
8 M. cremaster
9 Testes covered by the internal spermatic fascia
10 Caudoventral blind sac covered by the superficial sheet of the greater omentum
11 Left ventral coronary groove covered by the superficial sheet of the greater omentum
12 Ventral sac of the rumen covered by the superficial sheet of the greater omentum
13 Body of the abomasum
14 Apex of the heart

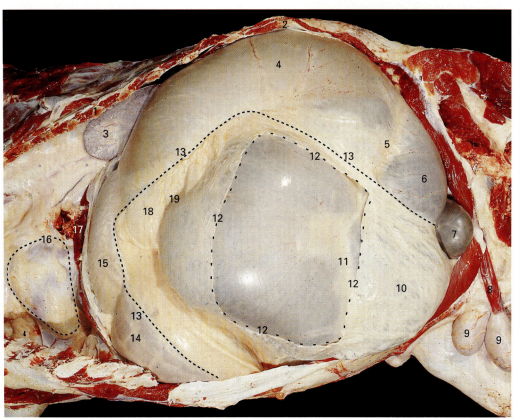

268. The bovine stomach *in situ* seen from the left side.

1 Rib 8
2 Rib 13
3 Spleen, reflected
4 Dorsal sac of the rumen
5 Left dorsal coronary groove
6 Dorsal caudal blind sac
7 Apex of the caecum
8 M. cremaster
9 Testes covered by the internal spermatic fascia
10 Caudoventral blind sac covered by the superficial sheet of the greater omentum
11 Left ventral coronary groove
12 Window cut in the superficial sheet of the greater omentum to reveal the ventral sac of the rumen
13 Line of attachment of the greater omentum as seen on the left. It comes into view in the caudal groove, passes cranially along the left longitudinal groove, then crosses the atrium of the rumen to reach the greater curvature of the abomasum
14 Body of the abomasum
15 Reticulum
16 Outline of the heart
17 Diaphragm
18 Atrium of the rumen
19 Cranial groove

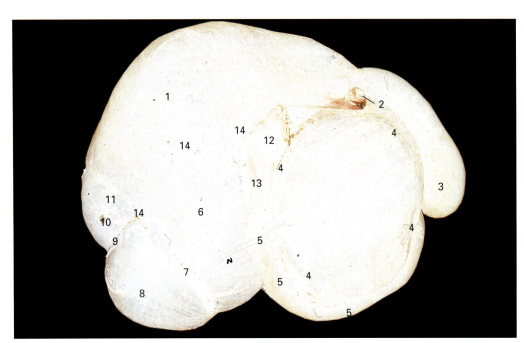

269. The stomach of a one-year-old bull seen from the right side.

1	Dorsal sac of the rumen	9	Caudal groove
2	Oesophagus	10	Caudodorsal blind sac
3	Reticulum	11	Right dorsal coronary groove
4	Omasum		
5	Abomasum	12	Beginning of the duodenum
6	Ventral sac of the rumen		
7	Right ventral coronary groove	13	Pylorus
		14	Right longitudinal groove
8	Caudoventral blind sac		

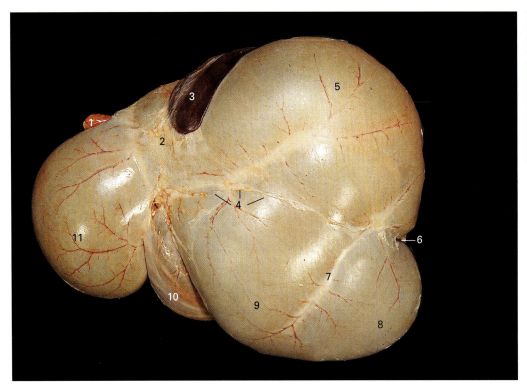

270. The stomach and spleen of a sheep seen from the left side. The omenta have been removed.

1	Oesophagus	7	Left ventral coronary groove
2	Atrium of the rumen		
3	Parietal surface of the spleen	8	Caudoventral blind sac
		9	Ventral sac of the rumen
4	Left longitudinal groove	10	Abomasum
5	Dorsal sac of the rumen	11	Reticulum
6	Caudal groove		

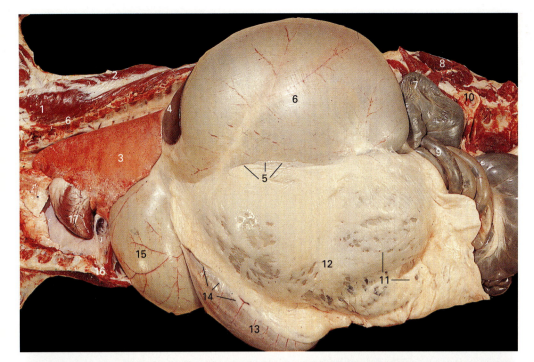

271. Left view of the contents of the thorax and abdomen of a sheep. The body wall has been removed and the diaphragm has been allowed to slip out of sight between the stomach and the left lung. The stomach is distended with gas which allows its compartments to be clearly distinguished but increases its size: this effect has been exaggerated by foreshortening.

1 M. longissimus thoracis	11 Superficial sheet of the greater omentum
2 M. rhomboideus cervicis	12 Ventral sac of the rumen covered by the superficial sheet of the greater omentum
3 Caudal lobe of the left lung	
4 Parietal surface of the spleen	
5 Left longitudinal groove of the rumen and the attachment of the greater omentum	13 Body of the abomasum
	14 Attachment of the superficial sheet of the greater omentum along the greater curvature of the abomasum
6 Dorsal sac of the rumen	
7 Part of the proximal loop of the ascending colon	
8 M. gluteus medius	15 Reticulum
9 Parts of the spiral loop of the ascending colon	16 Xiphisternal cartilage cut longitudinally
10 Acetabulum	17 Left ventricle

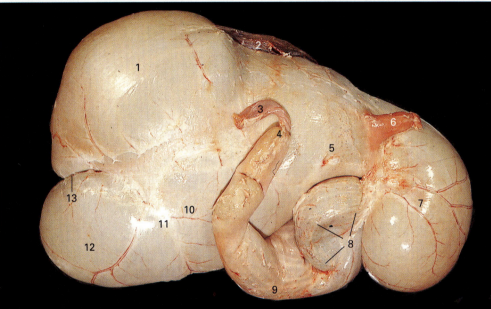

272. Right view of the stomach and spleen of a sheep. The omenta have been removed.

1 Dorsal sac of the rumen	8 Omasum
2 Dorsal end of the spleen	9 Body of the abomasum
3 Beginning of the descending duodenum	10 Ventral sac of the rumen
4 Pylorus	11 Right ventral coronary groove
5 Atrium of the rumen	12 Caudoventral blind sac
6 Oesophagus	13 Caudal groove
7 Reticulum	

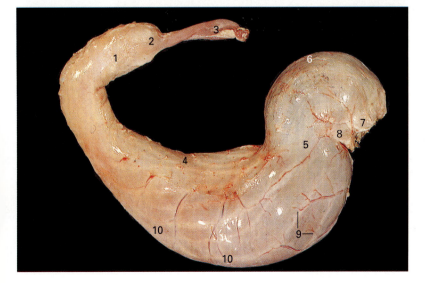

273. Left view of the omasum and abomasum of a sheep. The omenta have been removed.

1 Pyloric part of the abomasum	7 Position of the reticulo-omasal orifice
2 Pylorus	8 Lesser curvature of the omasum
3 Beginning of the descending duodenum	
4 Lesser curvature of the abomasum	9 Pale lines marking the attachments of the permanent mucosal folds on the inner surface
5 Position of the omaso-abomasal orifice	
6 Greater curvature of the omasum	10 Greater curvature of the abomasum

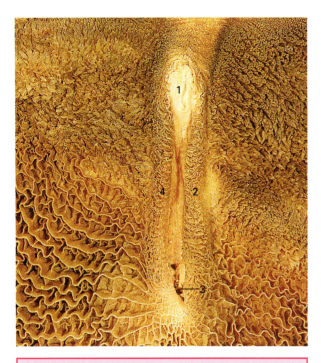

274. The reticular groove of a cow. The normal twist in the groove was obliterated when the structure was placed on a flat surface.

1 Cardia	3 Reticulo-omasal orifice
2 Right lip	4 Left lip

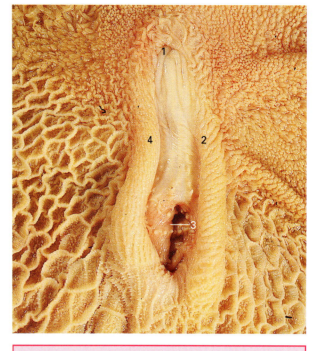

275. The reticular groove of a sheep. The normal twist in the groove was obliterated when the structure was placed on a flat surface.

1 Cardia	3 Reticulo-omasal orifice
2 Right lip	4 Left lip

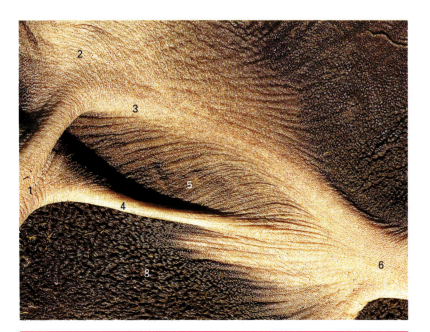

276. The interior of the right wall of the rumen of a one-year-old bull.

1 Cranial pillar	5 Island of the rumen (insula ruminis)
2 Dorsal sac with short villi	6 Caudal pillar
3 Accessory part of the right pillar	7 Beginning of the right ventral coronary pillar
4 Right pillar	8 Ventral sac with long villi

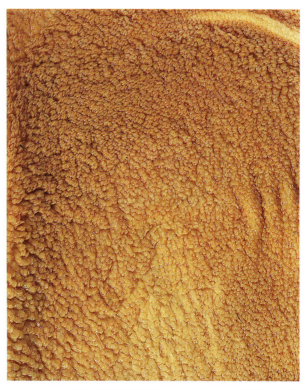

277. The mucosa of the ventral sac of the rumen of a sheep.

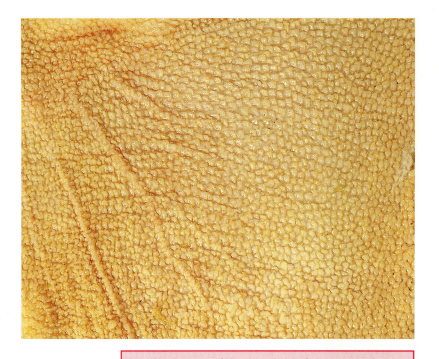

278. The mucosa of the dorsal sac of the rumen of a sheep.

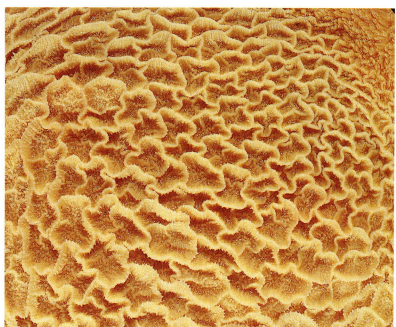

279. The mucosa of the reticulum of a sheep. The area shown is the most ventral part of the organ.

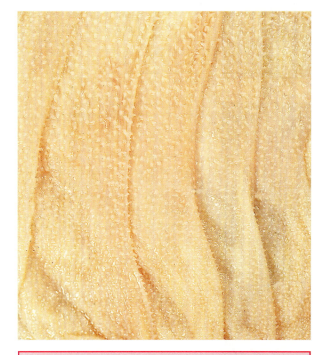

280. The mucosa of the omasum of a sheep. The greater curvature is to the left and the lesser curvature to the right. Moving from left to right, the edges of progressively larger mucosal folds can be seen.

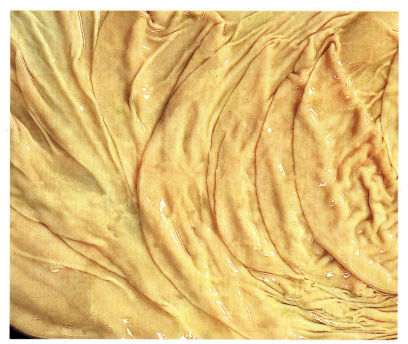

281. The mucosa of the abomasum of a sheep showing some of the permanent folds.

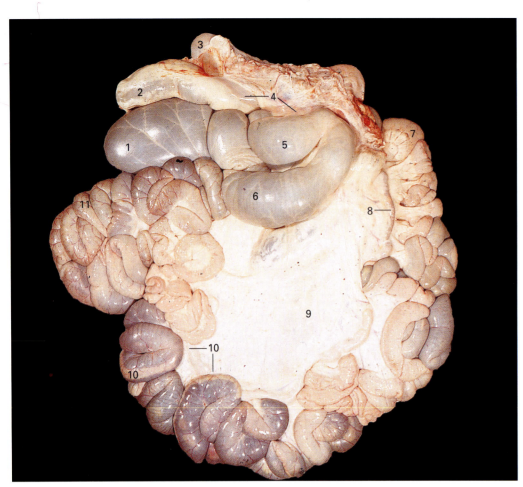

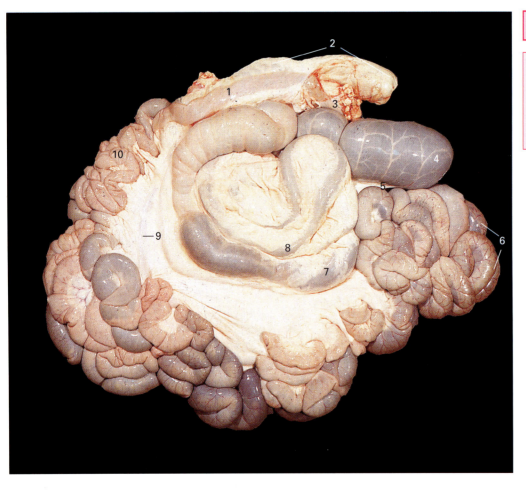

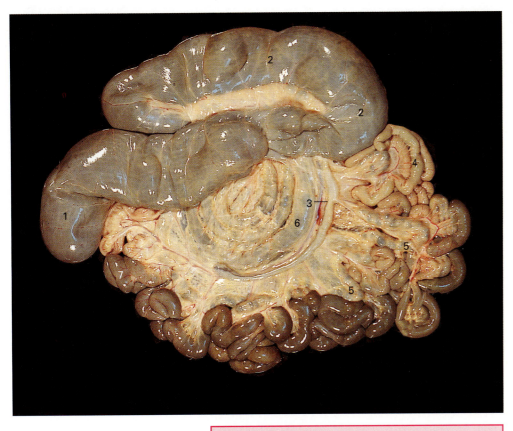

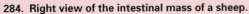

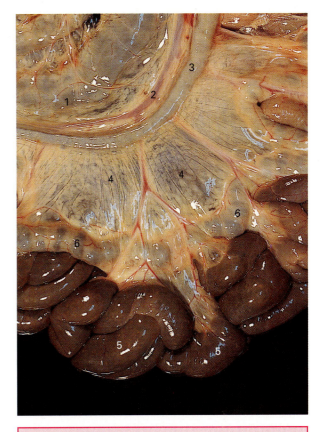

284. Right view of the intestinal mass of a sheep.

1 Apex of the caecum
2 The initial part of the proximal loop of the ascending colon
3 A mesenteric lymph node
4 Proximal part of jejunum
5 Outermost centrifugal coil of the spiral loop
6 Outermost centripetal coil of the spiral loop
7 Distal part of the jejunum

285. Detail of the intestinal mass of a sheep seen from the right side.

1 Part of the outermost centripetal coil of the spiral loop
2 Mesenteric veins; the accompanying arteries are devoid of blood and not easily seen
3 Part of a mesenteric lymph node
4 Mesentery containing a little fat; the fine radial lines are lymphatics
5 Jejunum
6 Part of the outermost centrifugal coil of the spiral loop

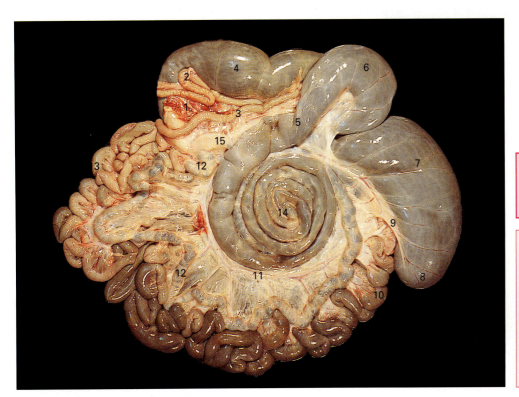

286. Left view of the intestinal mass of a sheep. The transverse colon and the descending colon were retained within the abdomen and are not seen in the specimen.

1 Cut root of the mesentery
2 Ascending duodenum
3 Descending duodenum
4 Proximal loop of the ascending colon
5 Beginning of the outermost centripetal coil of the spiral loop
6 Terminal part of the proximal loop of the ascending colon
7 Body of the caecum
8 Apex of the caecum
9 Free edge of the ileocaecal fold
10 Distal part of the jejunum
11 Mesenteric vessels
12 Outermost centrifugal coil of the spiral loop
13 Proximal part of the jejunum
14 Centre of the spiral loop of the ascending colon
15 Beginning of the distal loop of the ascending colon

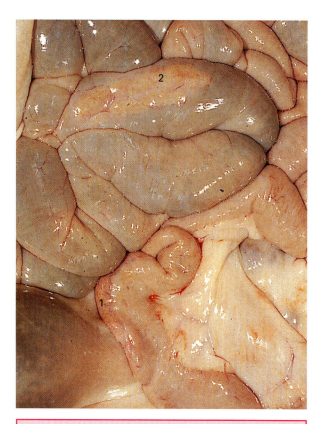

287. Loops of bovine small intestine showing aggregated lymphatic nodules (Peyer's patches) in (1) contracted and (2) relaxed segments.

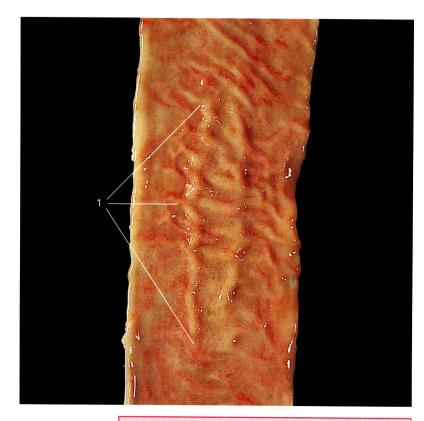

288. The mucosal surface of a section of the bovine jejunum opened along the mesenteric side showing (1) an aggregated lymphatic nodule (Peyer's patch).

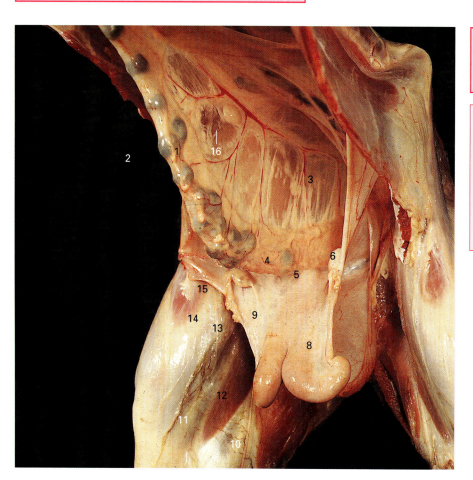

289. Left ventral view of the caudal abdominal and pelvic viscera of a ewe seen after removal of the body wall and most of the abdominal contents. The carcass is suspended as if in the standing position.

1 Mesocolon	10 M. gracilis
2 Descending colon	11 M. sartorius
3 Free edge of the left broad ligament of the uterus	12 Middle of the right horn of the uterus
4 Beginning of the rectum	13 Right broad ligament
5 Left ovary	14 Coils of the uterine tube (oviduct)
6 Lateral ligament of the bladder	15 Right ovary with a medium-sized ovarian follicle
7 M. tensor fasciae latae	
8 Bladder	16 Caudal mesenteric vein
9 Body of the uterus	

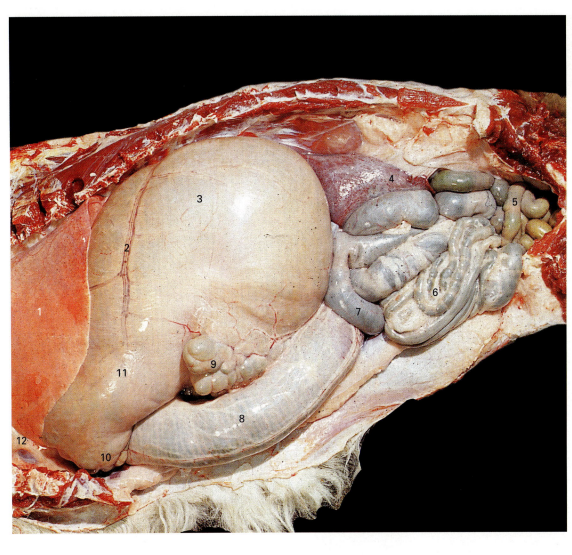

290. Left view of the caudal thoracic and abdominal contents of a llama *in situ*. The left body wall has been removed; the cut edge of the diaphragm is concealed between the lung and stomach.

1 Caudal lobe of the left lung
2 Branches of the coeliac artery and portal vein
3 First compartment of the stomach
4 Spleen
5 Loops of jejunum
6 Spiral part of the ascending colon
7 Wide proximal part of the ascending colon
8 Third compartment of the stomach covered by the semitransparent greater omentum
9 Caudal group of glandular saccules
10 Cranial group of glandular saccules, just visible in profile
11 Cranioventral part of the first compartment of the stomach
12 Pericardium

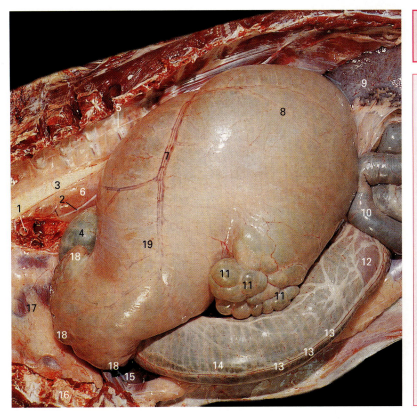

291. A llama stomach and related structures *in situ* seen from the left side. The diaphragm has been removed.

1 Cut left principal bronchus
2 Dorsal trunk of the left vagus nerve
3 Aorta
4 Proximal end of the third compartment
5 Sympathetic trunk
6 Oesophagus
7 Branches of the coeliac artery and portal vein
8 Caudal sac of the first compartment
9 Spleen
10 Wide proximal part of the ascending colon
11 Glandular saccules of the caudal sac of the first compartment
12 Terminal part of the third compartment with its distinctive colour provided by the true gastric glands
13 Line of attachment of the greater omentum
14 Middle part of the third compartment seen through the semitransparent greater omentum
15 Liver
16 Cut costal cartilages 6 and 7
17 Pericardium covering the heart
18 Glandular saccules of the cranial sac of the first compartment, seen in profile
19 Cranial sac of the first compartment

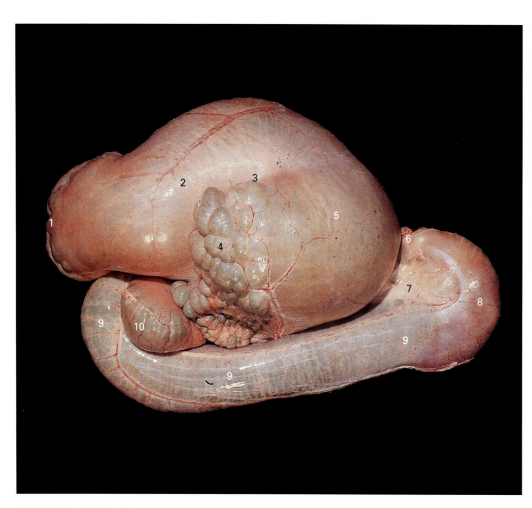

292. Left view of the stomach of a llama. It is somewhat dilated by gastric gas.

1 Glandular saccules of the cranial sac of the first compartment, seen in profile
2 Cranial sac of the first compartment
3 Left end of the groove separating the cranial and caudal sacs of the first compartment
4 Glandular saccules of the caudal sac of the first compartment
5 Caudal sac of the first compartment
6 Pylorus
7 Lesser omentum attached to the lesser curvature of the preterminal flexure of the third compartment
8 Terminal part of the third compartment lined by proper gastric glands
9 Part of the third compartment with a mucous lining but no proper gastric glands
10 Second compartment

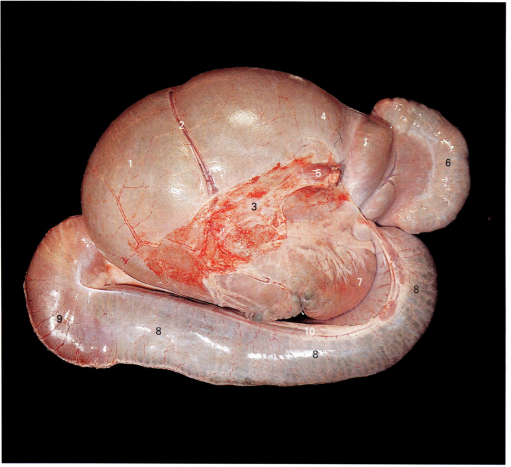

293. Right view of the stomach of a llama. It is somewhat dilated by gastric gas.

1 Caudal sac of the first compartment
2 Branches of the coeliac artery and the portal vein
3 Area of attachment to the left abdominal roof
4 Cranial sac of the first compartment
5 Cardia and the terminal part of the oesophagus
6 Glandular saccules of the cranial sac of the first compartment seen in profile
7 Second compartment
8 Part of the third compartment with a mucous lining but no proper gastric glands
9 Terminal part of the third compartment lined by true gastric glands; the pyloric region of the stomach has been tucked behind the caudal sac of the first compartment to give a better view of the latter structure
10 Line of attachment of the lesser omentum

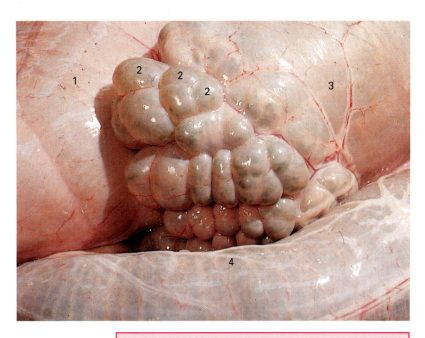

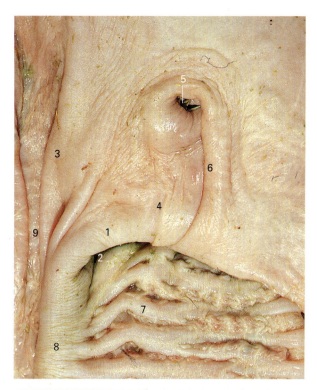

294. Detail of the glandular saccules of the caudal sac of the first compartment of a llama stomach seen from the serosal surface.

1 Cranial sac of the first compartment	3 Caudal sac of the first compartment
2 Glandular saccules	4 Middle part of the third compartment

295. The mucosal surface of a llama stomach showing the cardia, the gastric groove and some of the glandular saccules of the caudal sac of the first compartment. The top of the photograph is craniodorsal.

1 Caudal branch of the transverse pillar	6 Muscular lip of the gastric groove
2 Opening from the first to the second compartment	7 Glandular saccules of the caudal sac of the first compartment
3 Cranial branch of the transverse pillar	8 Transverse pillar
4 Membranous lip of the gastric groove	9 Mucosa of the cranial sac of the first compartment
5 Cardia	

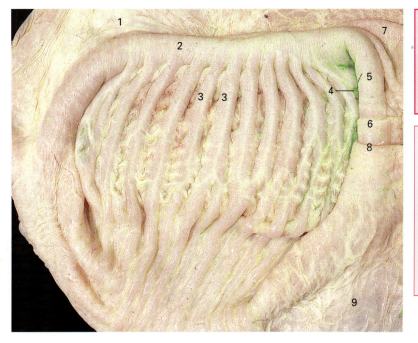

296. The mucosal surface of a llama stomach showing the saccules of the caudal sac of the first compartment. The top of the photograph is craniodorsal. (Initially this would seem to conflict with the orientation of the previous photograph but because the structures are curved, both statements are reasonable approximations.)

1 Mucosa of the cranial sac of the first compartment	5 Caudal branch of the transverse pillar
2 Transverse pillar separating the ventral parts of the cranial and caudal sacs of the first compartment	6 Membranous lip of the gastric groove
3 Primary crests separating the saccules. The secondary crests pass between the primary crests and are perpendicular to them	7 Cranial branch of the transverse pillar
	8 Muscular lip of the gastric groove
4 Opening from the first to the second compartment	9 Mucosa of the caudal sac of the first compartment

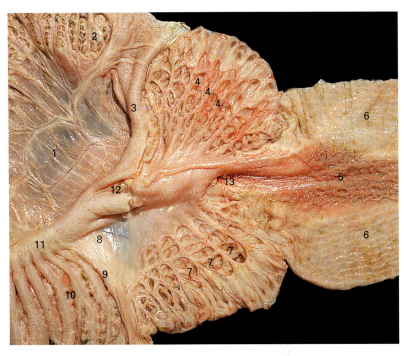

297. The mucosal surface of the second gastric compartment of a llama. The organ was opened along its greater curvature and is continuous with the first compartment on the left and third compartment on the right.

1 Mucosa of the cranial sac of the first compartment
2 Glandular saccules of the cranial sac of the first compartment
3 Cranial branch of the transverse pillar
4 Glandular cells of the cranial wall of the second compartment
5 Part of the mucosa of the third compartment bearing reticular mucosal pleats
6 Part of the mucosa of the third compartment bearing longitudinal mucosal pleats
7 Glandular cells of the caudal wall of the second compartment
8 Position of the opening from the first to the second compartment
9 Most craniodorsal of the primary crests related to the glandular saccules of the caudal sac of the first compartment
10 Glandular saccules of the caudal sac of the first compartment
11 Transverse pillar
12 Cut caudal branch of the transverse pillar
13 Position of the opening from the second to the third compartment

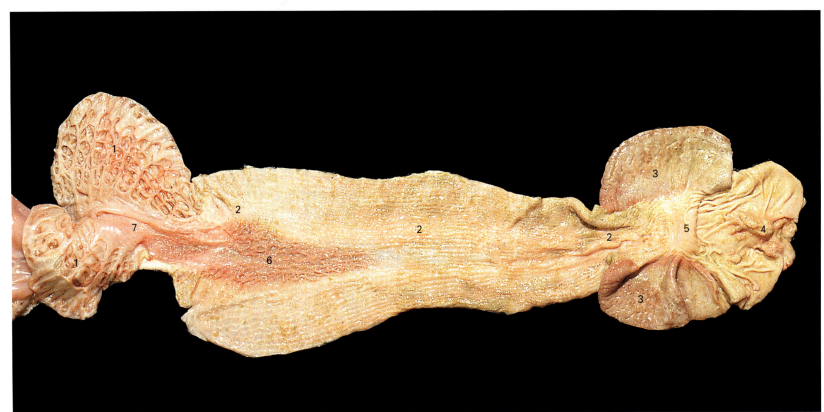

298. The second and third compartments of a llama stomach opened along the greater curvature.

1 Second compartment
2 Part of the mucosa of the third compartment bearing numerous longitudinal mucosal pleats
3 Part of the mucosa of the third compartment bearing proper gastric glands
4 Torus of the pylorus
5 Position of the preterminal flexure
6 Part of the mucosa of the third compartment bearing reticular mucosal pleats
7 Continuation of the gastric groove within the second compartment

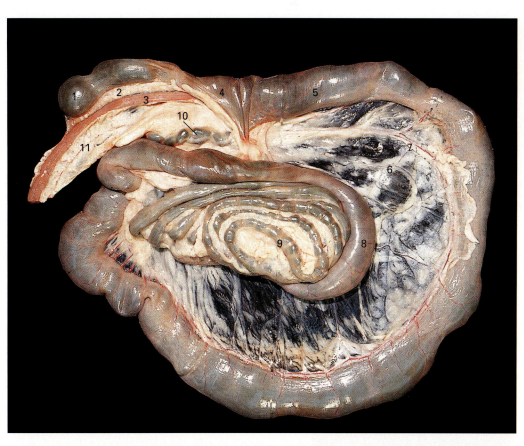

299. Right view of the ileum and ascending colon of a llama after being laid flat. Contrary to expectation, the mesocolon of the outer coil and the central spiral are not adherent.

1 Apex of the caecum	8 First centripetal coil of the
2 Ileocaecal fold	spiral colon
3 Terminal part of the ileum	9 Junction of the centripetal
4 Caecocolic junction	and centrifugal coils
5 Proximal part of the	10 Beginning of the
ascending colon	transverse colon
6 Mesocolon	11 Part of the mesentery
7 Colic vessels	

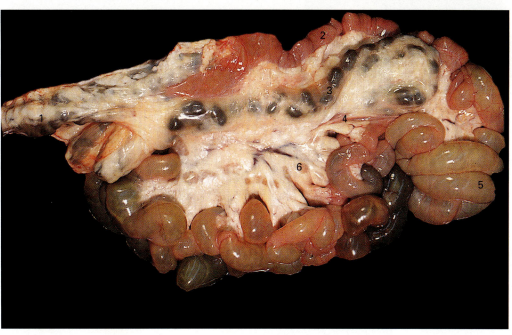

300. Part of the small intestine of a llama showing parts of the descending colon embedded in the base of the mesentery.

1 Beginning of the rectum	4 Mesenteric vessels
2 Descending duodenum	5 Jejunum
3 Part of the descending	6 Mesenteric lymph nodes
colon fused to the	
mesentery	

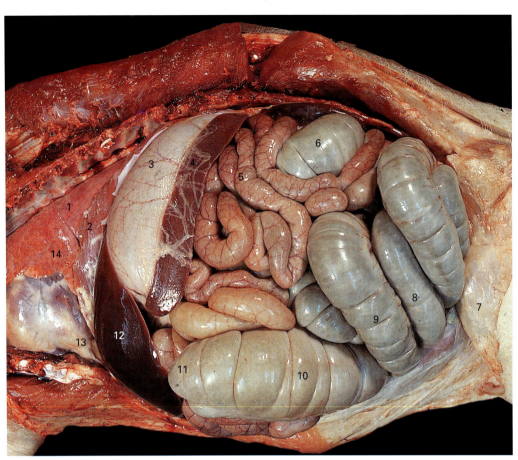

1 Caudal lobe of the left lung	8 Centrifugal coil of the ascending colon
2 Costal part of the diaphragm reflected cranially	9 Centripetal coil of the ascending colon
3 Stomach	10 Body of the caecum
4 Spleen, partially covered on its parietal surface by a fold of the greater omentum	11 Apex of the caecum
	12 Left lateral lobe of the liver
5 Loops of small intestine	13 Apex of the heart seen through the pericardium
6 Part of the first centripetal coil of the ascending colon	14 Caudal division of the cranial lobe of the left lung
7 Stifle joint	

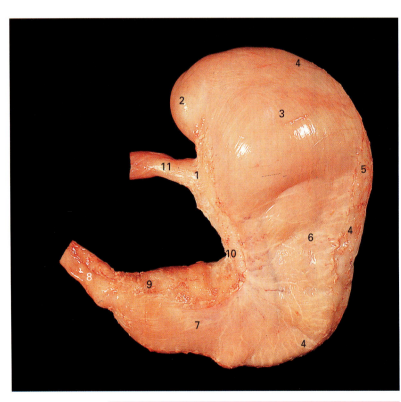

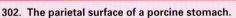

302. The parietal surface of a porcine stomach.

1 Cardia	7 Pyloric region
2 Diverticulum	8 Pylorus
3 Fundus	9 Line of attachment of the lesser omentum
4 Greater curvature	
5 Line of attachment of the greater omentum	10 Lesser curvature
	11 Oesophagus
6 Body of the stomach	

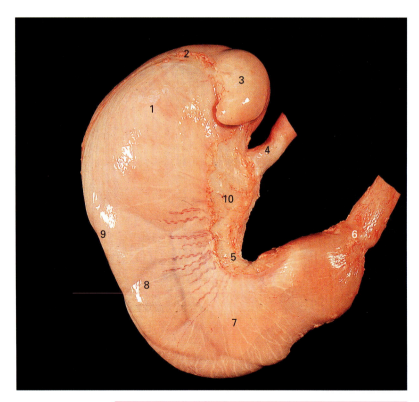

303. The visceral surface of a porcine stomach.

1 Fundus	7 Pyloric region
2 Line of attachment of the greater omentum	8 Body of the stomach
3 Diverticulum	9 Greater curvature
4 Oesophagus	10 Line of attachment of the lesser omentum
5 Lesser curvature	
6 Pylorus	

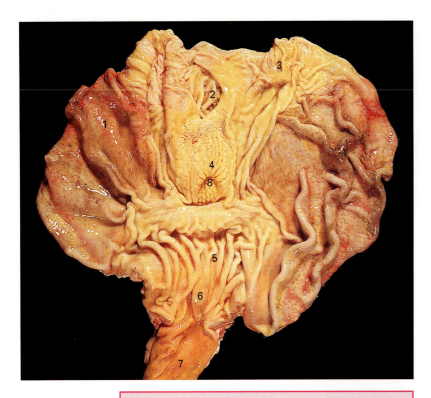

304. The mucosal surface of a porcine stomach. The organ has been opened along the greater curvature.

1	Gastric gland region	5	Pyloric gland region
2	Diverticulum	6	Pyloric torus lying within
3	Cardiac gland region		the pyloric opening
4	Area of cornified	7	Duodenal mucosa
	epithelium surrounding	8	Cardia
	the cardia		

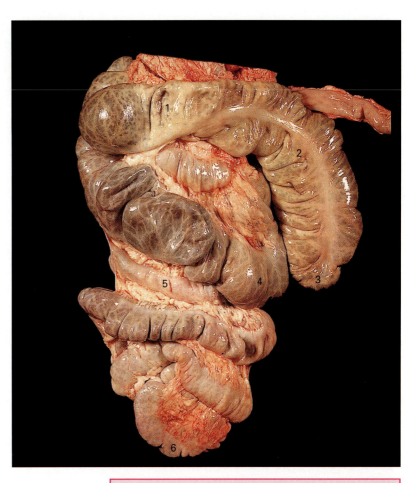

306. The spiral ascending colon of a pig seen from the left side. The structure can rotate somewhat about its axis but this is a common orientation.

1	Position where the caecum	3	Apex of the caecum
	and ascending colon	4	First centripetal coil
	merge	5	Adjacent centrifugal coil
2	Body of the caecum	6	Apex of the spiral colon

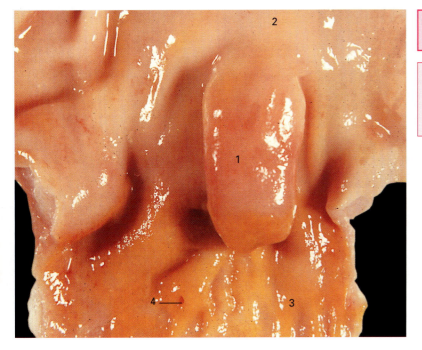

305. Detail of the mucosa of the pyloric region of a porcine stomach.

1	Pyloric torus	4	Opening of the bile duct
2	Pyloric gland region of the		on the major duodenal
	stomach		papilla
3	Duodenal mucosa stained		
	with bile		

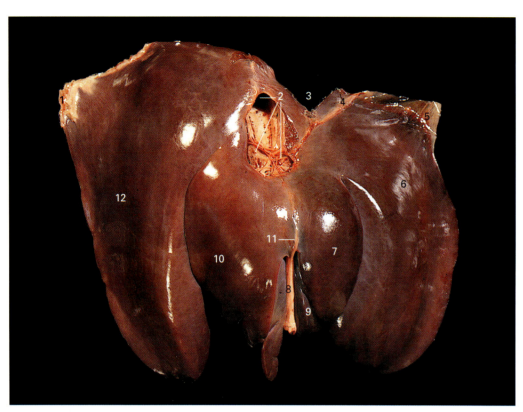

307. The parietal surface of the liver of a four-month-old foal.

1 Right triangular ligament	7 Left medial lobe
2 Caudal vena cava passing cranioventrally through the liver; numerous hepatic veins of various sizes can be seen joining it	8 Falciform ligament containing the remnant of the umbilical vein in its free edge
3 Oesophageal notch	9 Quadrate lobe
4 Left coronary ligament	10 Right medial lobe
5 Left triangular ligament	11 Line of attachment of the falciform ligament
6 Left lateral lobe	12 Right lateral lobe

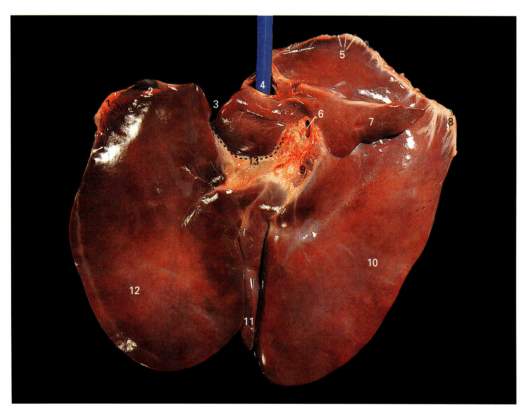

308. The visceral surface of the liver of a four-month-old foal. A blue plastic rod has been inserted into the caudal vena cava to make its position clear.

1 Left triangular ligament	8 Right triangular ligament
2 Left coronary ligament	9 Hepatic lymph nodes at the porta of the liver
3 Oesophageal notch	10 Right lateral lobe
4 Caudal vena cava	11 Quadrate lobe
5 Right coronary ligament	12 Left lateral lobe
6 Portal vein entering the liver	13 Line of attachment of the lesser omentum
7 Caudate lobe	

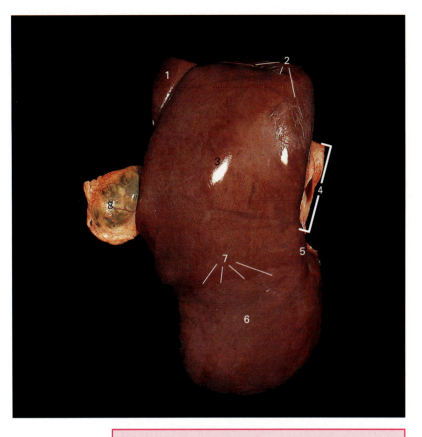

309. The diaphragmatic surface of the bovine liver.

1 Caudate lobe	5 Oesophageal notch
2 Line of attachment of the coronary ligament	6 Left lobe
3 Right lobe	7 Line of attachment of the falciform ligament
4 Caudal vena cava	8 Gall bladder

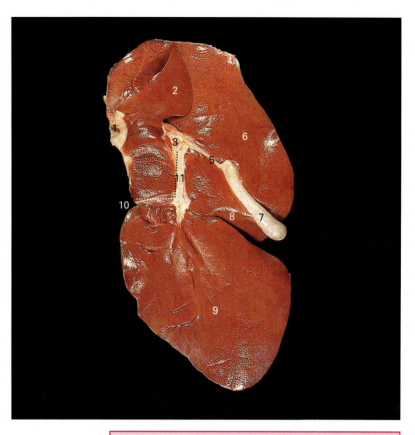

311. The visceral surface of the liver of a sheep.

1 Caudal vena cava	7 Gall bladder
2 Caudate lobe	8 Quadrate lobe
3 Porta of the liver	9 Left lobe
4 Right triangular ligament	10 Oesophageal notch
5 Cystic duct	11 Line of attachment of the lesser omentum
6 Right lobe	

310. The diaphragmatic surface of the liver of a sheep.

1 Right triangular ligament	6 Line of attachment of the falciform ligament
2 Coronary ligament	7 Left lobe
3 Area of the liver adherent to the diaphragm	8 Gall bladder
4 Caudal vena cava	9 Right lobe
5 Oesphageal notch	

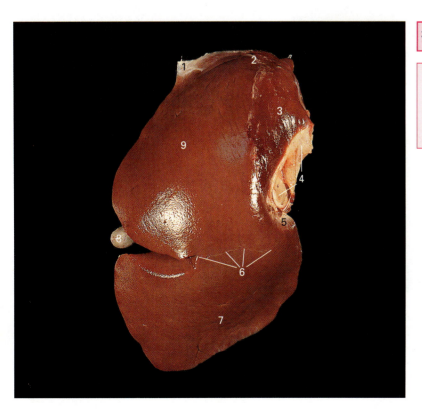

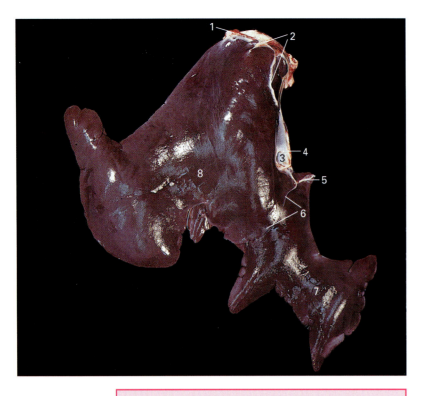

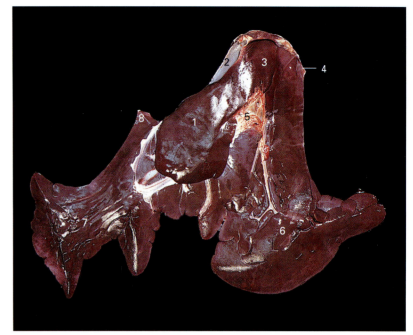

313. Visceral surface of the liver of a llama.

312. Diaphragmatic surface of the liver of a llama.

1	Right triangular ligament	5	Left coronary ligament
2	Right coronary ligament	6	Falciform ligament
3	Openings of the hepatic veins	7	Left lobe
4	Caudal vena cava	8	Right lobe

1	Papillary process of caudate lobe	6	Right lobe
2	Caudal vena cava	7	Left lobe
3	Caudate process of caudate lobe	8	Left triangular ligament
4	Right triangular ligament	9	Line of attachment of the lesser omentum, partially hidden by the caudate process
5	Porta		

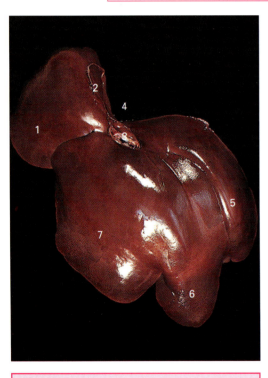

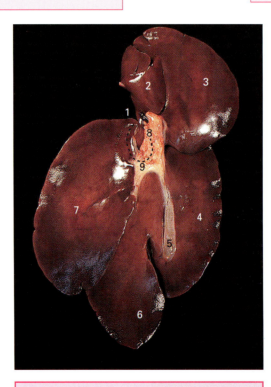

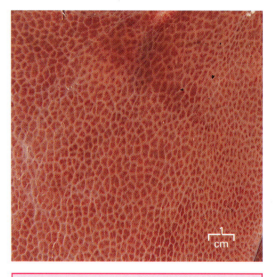

316. Detail showing the texture of the surface of a pig's liver. Each lobule is surrounded by a distinct layer of connective tissue.

314. The parietal surface of the liver of a pig.

315. The visceral surface of the liver of a pig.

1	Right lateral lobe	4	Oesophageal notch
2	Caudal vena cava	5	Left lateral lobe
3	Hepatic veins entering the caudal vena cava	6	Left medial lobe
		7	Right medial lobe

1	Oesophageal notch	6	Left medial lobe
2	Caudate lobe	7	Left lateral lobe
3	Right lateral lobe	8	Porta
4	Right medial lobe	9	Line of attachment of the lesser omentum
5	Gall bladder		

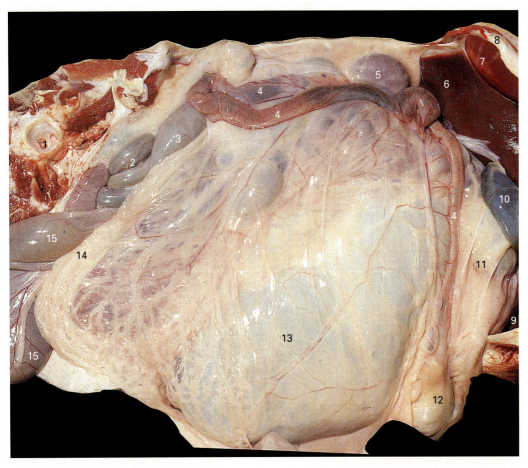

317. The abdominal contents of a sheep seen from the right side. The body wall has been removed.

1 Acetabulum
2 Loops of jejunum
3 Part of the proximal loop of the ascending colon
4 Descending duodenum
5 Right kidney
6 Right lobe of the liver
7 Abdominal surface of the diaphragm
8 Caudal border of the rib cage
9 Left lobe of the liver
10 Gall bladder
11 Lesser omentum
12 Pyloric part of the abomasum
13 Ventral sac of the rumen seen through the superficial sheet of the greater omentum
14 Line of reflection of the omentum where the superficial and deep sheets are continuous with one another
15 Caecum

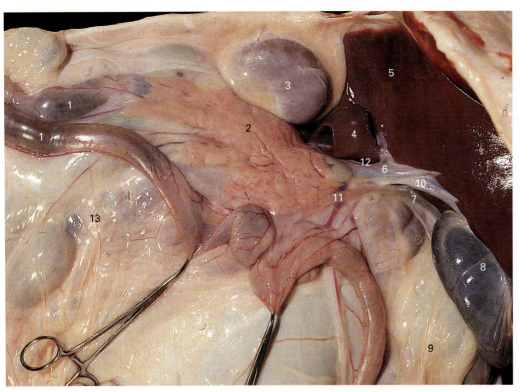

318. Right view of the pancreas and related structures in a sheep.

1 Descending duodenum
2 Pancreas
3 Right kidney
4 Caudate lobe of the liver
5 Visceral surface of the right lobe of the liver
6 Portal vein
7 Bile duct
8 Gall bladder
9 Lesser omentum
10 Cystic duct
11 Common bile duct
12 Omental (epiploic) foramen
13 Superficial sheet of the greater omentum

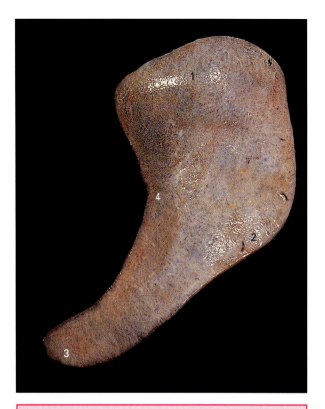

319. Parietal surface of the spleen of a horse.

1 Dorsal end	3 Ventral end
2 Caudal border	4 Cranial border

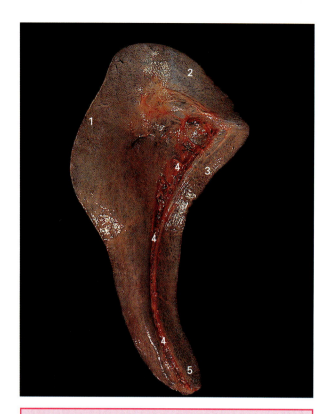

320. Visceral surface of the spleen of a horse.

1 Caudal border	4 Hilus
2 Dorsal end	5 Ventral end
3 Cranial border	

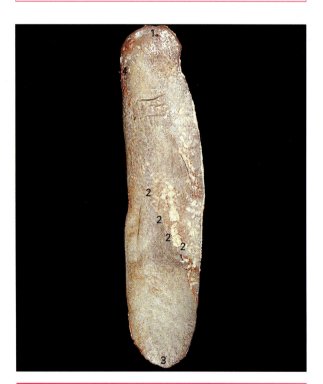

321. Parietal surface of the bovine spleen.

1 Dorsal end	3 Ventral end
2 Line of peritoneal reflection; the area ventral to this line has a peritoneal covering	4 The hilus is close to this point on the visceral surface

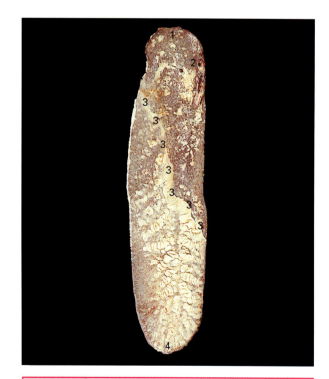

322. Visceral surface of the bovine spleen.

1 Dorsal end	3 Line of peritoneal reflection; the area ventral to this line has a peritoneal covering
2 Hilus	
	4 Ventral end

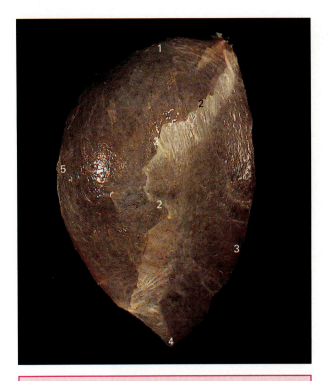

323. Parietal surface of the spleen of a sheep.

1 Dorsal end	3 Caudal border
2 Line of peritoneal reflection; the area ventral to this line has a peritoneal covering	4 Ventral end
	5 Cranial border

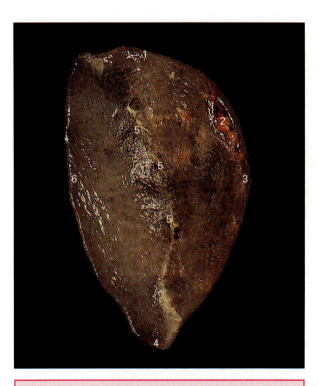

324. Visceral surface of the spleen of a sheep.

1 Dorsal end	5 Line of peritoneal
2 Hilus	reflection; the area ventral
3 Cranial border	to this line has a
4 Ventral end	peritoneal covering
	6 Caudal border

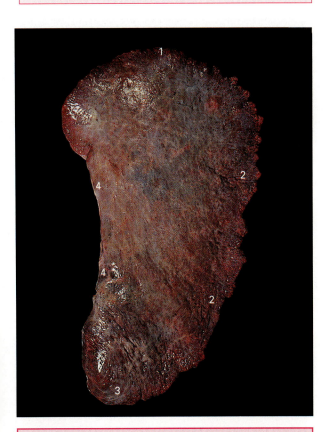

325. Parietal surface of the spleen of a llama.

1 Dorsal end	3 Ventral end
2 Caudal border	4 Cranial border

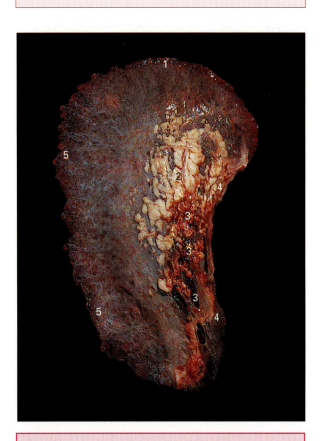

326. Visceral surface of the spleen of a llama.

1 Dorsal end	4 Cranial border
2 Subperitoneal fat	5 Caudal border
3 Hilus	

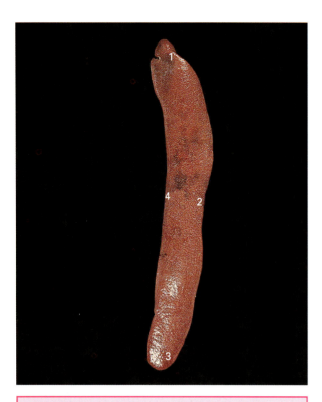

327. Parietal surface of the spleen of a pig.

1 Dorsal end	3 Ventral end
2 Caudal border	4 Cranial border

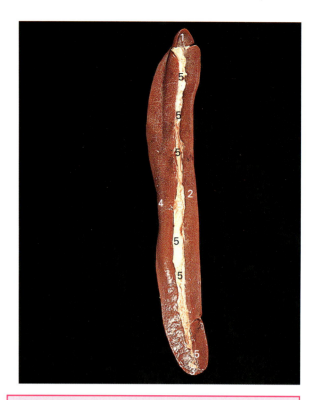

328. Visceral surface of the spleen of a pig.

1 Dorsal end	4 Caudal border
2 Gastric impression	5 Hilus
3 Ventral end	

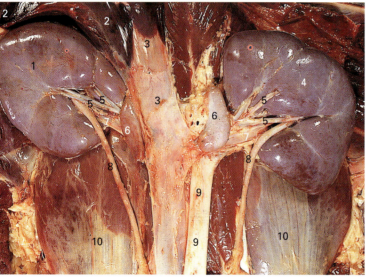

329. Ventral view of the kidneys and related structures in a horse.

1 Ventral surface of the right kidney	5 Renal arteries
2 Most caudal part of the caudate lobe of the liver	6 Adrenal gland
3 Caudal vena cava	7 Renal vein
4 Ventral surface of the left kidney	8 Ureter
	9 Aorta
	10 M. iliopsoas

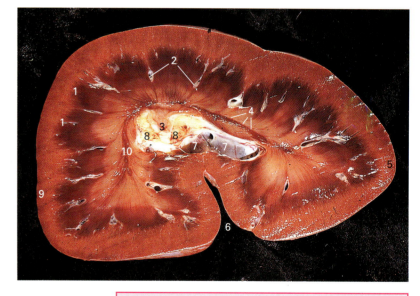

330. A dorsal section of the left kidney of a horse seen from the ventral aspect.

1 Corticomedullary junction	5 Caudal pole
2 Lobar vessels seen in section	6 Renal hilus
3 Mucosa lining the renal pelvis	7 Renal veins seen in section leaving the kidney
4 Terminal recess of the caudal pole surrounded by the pale striated tissue of the inner medulla	8 Fat lying in the renal sinus
	9 Cranial pole
	10 Terminal recess of the cranial pole

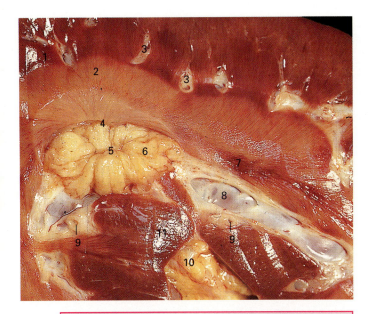

331. Detail of the pelvis of the kidney of a horse. The kidney is sectioned in the dorsal plane and is seen from the dorsal side.

1 Dark outer medulla
2 Pale inner medulla
3 Lobar vessels seen in section
4 Renal crest
5 Opening into the ureter
6 Mucosa of the medusa-like renal pelvis
7 Terminal recess seen in oblique section
8 Large renal vein in longitudinal section
9 Branch of the renal artery seen in section
10 Fat in the renal hilus
11 Part of the renal cortex adjacent to the renal hilus

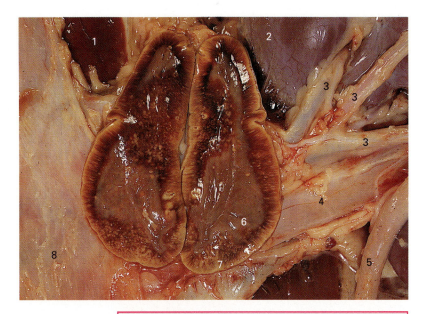

332. Dorsal section of the left adrenal gland of a horse. The ventral half of the gland has been reflected towards the animal's right (the left of the photograph) so that both halves are shown.

1 Part of the left crus of the diaphragm
2 Ventral surface of left kidney
3 Renal arteries
4 Renal vein
5 Ureter
6 Adrenal medulla
7 Adrenal cortex
8 Ventral surface of the caudal vena cava

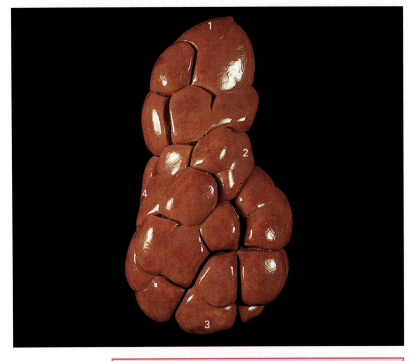

333. Left lateral view of the left bovine kidney with the perirenal fat and the renal capsule removed.

1 Cranial pole
2 Depression in the dorsal surface close to the hilus
3 Caudal pole
4 Ventral border

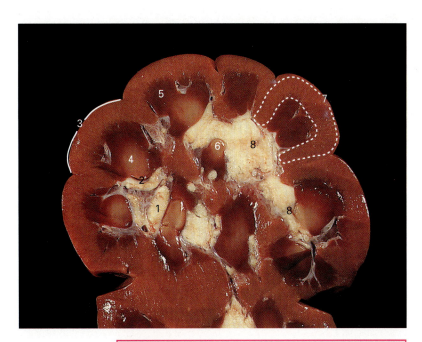

334. Dorsal section of one pole of a bovine kidney.

1 Fat occupying the renal sinus
2 Cavity of a minor calyx
3 A renal lobe
4 Pale inner medulla extending to the papilla
5 Dark outer medulla
6 A papilla tip
7 Renal cortex
8 Branches of the collecting system conducting urine from the minor calyces to the major calyx

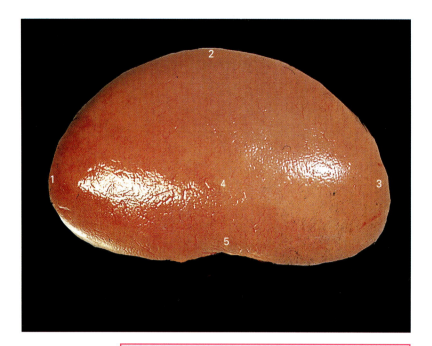

335. Dorsal view of the right kidney of a sheep. The renal capsule has been removed.

1 Cranial pole	4 Dorsal surface
2 Lateral border	5 Hilus
3 Caudal pole	

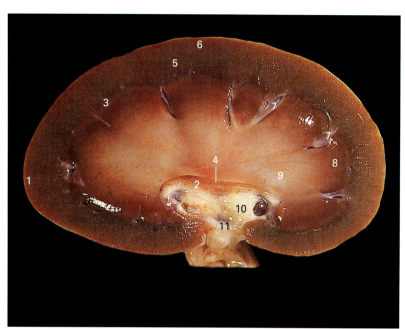

336. Dorsal section of the right kidney of a sheep seen from the dorsal aspect.

1 Cranial pole	7 Lobar vessels
2 Renal pelvis	8 Outer medulla
3 Corticomedullary junction	9 Inner medulla
4 Renal crest	10 Fat lying in the renal sinus
5 Cortex	11 Renal end of the ureter in
6 Lateral border	section

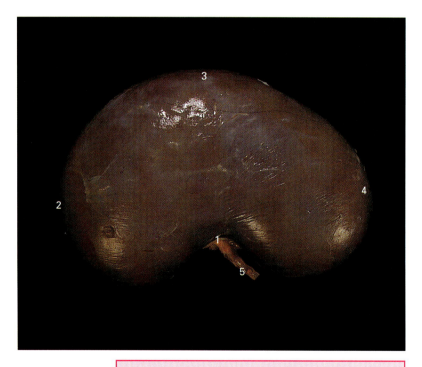

337. Dorsal view of the right kidney of a llama. The perirenal fat, but not the capsule, has been removed.

1 Hilus	4 Caudal pole
2 Cranial pole	5 Ureter
3 Lateral border	

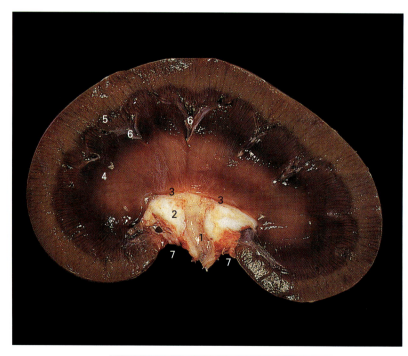

338. The right kidney of a llama in dorsal section.

1 Ureter	4 Junction of outer and
2 Fat contained in the renal	inner medulla
sinus	5 Corticomedullary junction
3 Renal crest	6 Lobar vessels
	7 Hilus

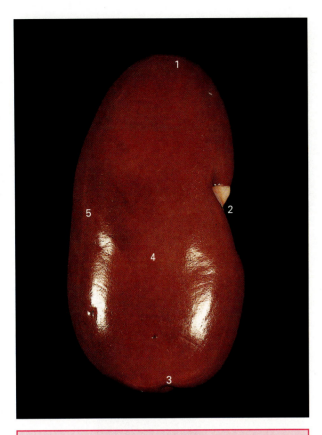

339. **Dorsal view of the left kidney of a pig with the capsule removed.**

1 Cranial pole	4 Dorsal surface
2 Hilus	5 Lateral border
3 Caudal pole	

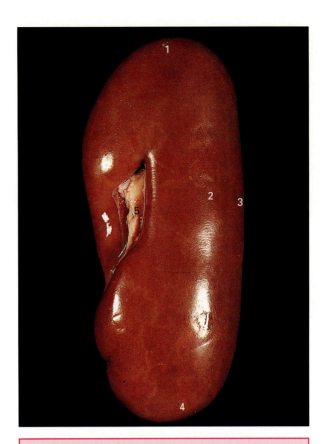

340. **Ventral view of the left kidney of a pig with the capsule removed.**

1 Cranial pole	4 Caudal pole
2 Ventral surface	5 Hilus
3 Lateral border	

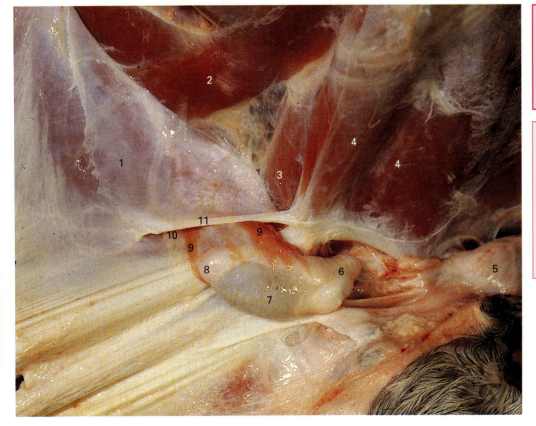

341. **The left inguinal region of a four-month-old colt. The skin has been removed and the penis and prepuce have been reflected caudally. The loose superficial connective tissue has been broken down by blunt dissection to show the superficial inguinal ring and related structures. Ventrolateral view. The left hand side of the photograph is cranial.**

1 Aponeurosis of the M. obliquus externus abdominis; the caudal muscular part of M. obliquus internus abdominis can be seen through it	6 Tail of the epididymis
	7 Testis seen through the intact internal spermatic fascia
	8 Head of the epididymis
2 M. sartorius	9 M. cremaster
3 M. pectineus	10 Superficial inguinal ring
4 M. gracilis	11 Ventral edge of the inguinal ligament (lateral crus of the superficial inguinal ring)
5 Body of the penis reflected caudally	

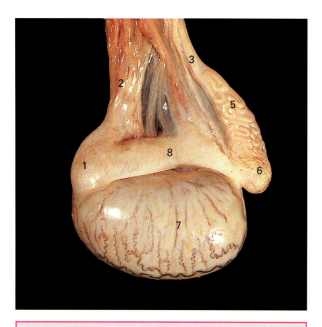

342. Lateral view of the left testis of a horse.

1 Head of the epididymis
2 Vascular cone of the testis;
   individual vessels cannot
   be seen through the
   connective tissue
3 Beginning of the straight
   part of the deferent duct
4 Mesorchium
5 Convoluted part of the
   deferent duct
6 Tail of the epididymis
7 Lateral surface of the testis
8 Body of the epididymis

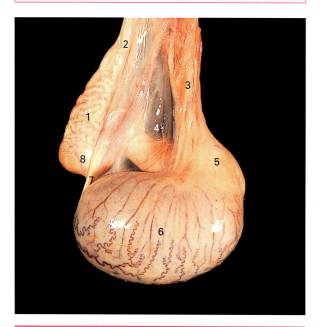

343. Medial view of the left testis of a horse.

1 Convoluted part of the
   deferent duct
2 Beginning of the straight
   part of the deferent duct
3 Vascular cone of the testis;
   individual vessels cannot
   be seen through the
   connective tissue
4 Mesorchium
5 Head of the epididymis
6 Medial surface of the
   testis
7 Ligament of the tail of the
   epididymis
8 Tail of the epididymis

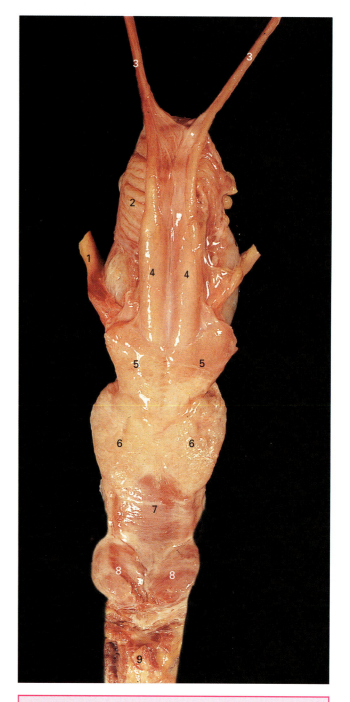

**344. Dorsal view of the bladder, pelvic urethra and
related structures in the stallion.**

1 Left ureter
2 Bladder, empty
3 Left and right deferent ducts
4 Ampullae
5 Left and right vesicular
   glands (seminal vesicles)
6 Left and right lobes of the
   prostate gland
7 Pelvic part of the urethra
   surrounded by the
   urethral muscle
8 Left and right bulbourethral
   glands enclosed in urethral
   muscle
9 Part of the bulb of the penis

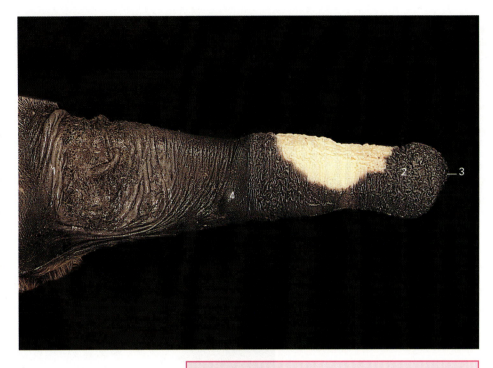

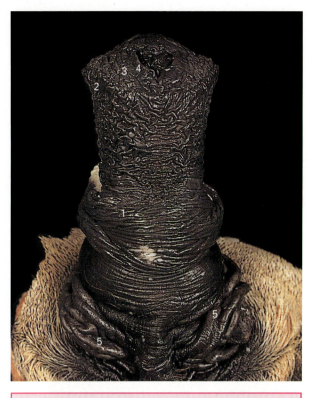

345. Right view of the free part of the penis of the horse. The prepuce has been everted. In this animal the penis had a large unpigmented area on its dorsal side.

1 Position of the preputial opening when the penis is retracted
2 Edge of the corona of the glans
3 Position of the urethral opening
4 Position of the preputial fold when the penis is retracted; it bears the vestigial nipple of the male

346. Ventral view of the free part of the penis of the horse. The prepuce is only partially everted.

1 Position of the preputial fold when the penis is retracted
2 Corona of the glans
3 Urethral process lying within the fossa glandis
4 Position of the urethral opening
5 Position of the preputial opening when the penis is retracted

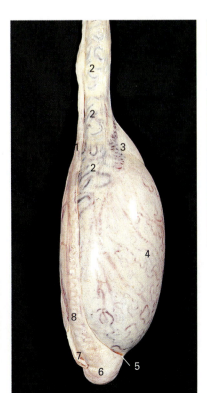

347. Caudomedial view of the left testis and related structures in a bull.

1 Beginning of the straight part of the deferent duct
2 Vascular cone of the testis
3 Head of the epididymis
4 Medial surface of the testis
5 Ligament of the tail of the epididymis
6 Tail of the epididymis
7 Cut scrotal ligament
8 Initial convoluted part of the deferent duct

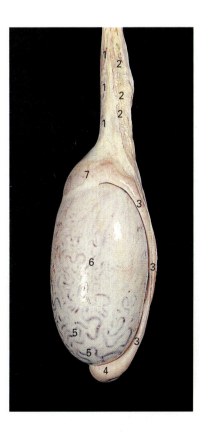

348. Lateral view of the left testis and related structures in a bull.

1 Vascular cone of the testis
2 Line of attachment of the mesofuniculus
3 Body of the epididymis
4 Tail of the epididymis
5 Superficial convoluted branches of the testicular artery
6 Testis enclosed in its dense fibrous capsule, the tunica albuginea
7 Head of the epididymis

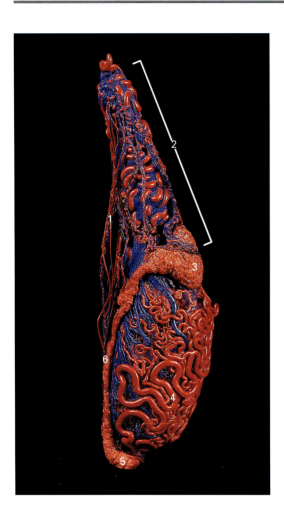

349. Lateral view of a cast of the blood vessels of the testis and related structures in a bull. All the tissues have been removed. The arteries are red and the veins blue.

1 Small vessels accompanying the deferent duct
2 Vascular cone consisting of the unbranched, but highly convoluted artery, and the delicate pampiniform venous plexus
3 Arteries of the head of the epididymis
4 Superficial convoluted branches of the testicular artery
5 Arteries of the tail of the epididymis
6 Arteries of the body of the epididymis

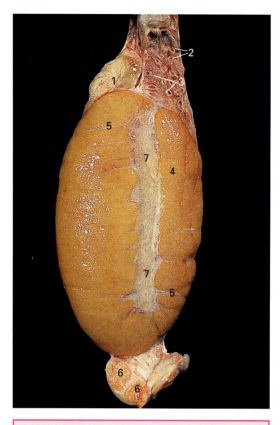

350. The testis of a bull sectioned in the sagittal plane.

1 Head of the epididymis
2 Highly convoluted testicular artery seen in section
3 Pampiniform plexus
4 Testicular parenchyma
5 Small fibrous septa supporting the testicular parenchyma
6 Tail of the epididymis
7 Mediastinum testis

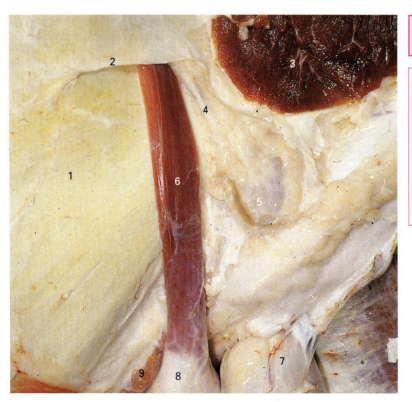

351. Lateral view of a superficial dissection of the left inguinal region of a bull.

1 Tunica flava
2 Ventral edge of the inguinal ligament (lateral crus of the superficial inguinal ring)
3 M. gracilis
4 External pudendal vessels
5 Superficial inguinal lymph node
6 M. cremaster; the spermatic cord lies on its medial surface
7 Part of the right testis
8 Dorsal end of the left testis; the internal spermatic fascia has been left in place and provides attachment for the M. cremaster
9 Part of M. praeputialis caudalis

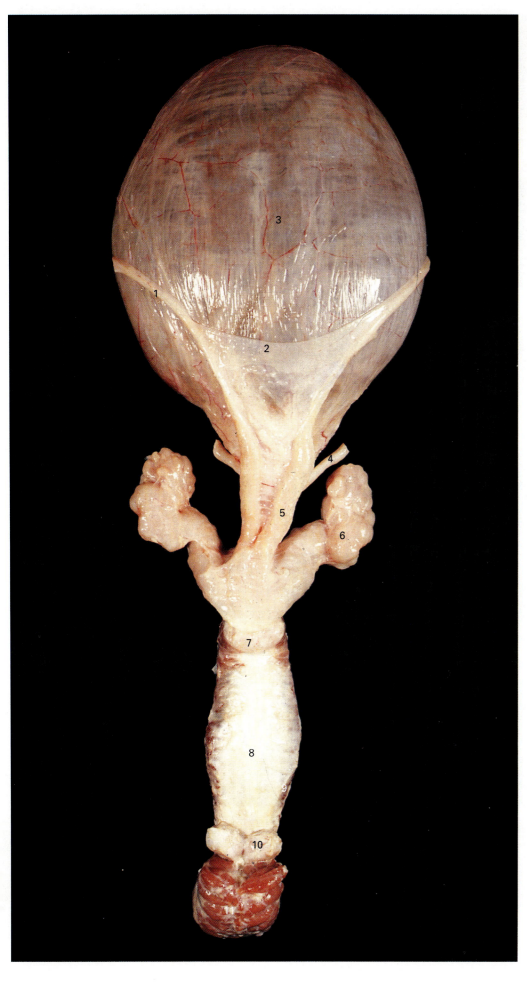

1 Left deferent duct	7 Body of the prostate gland
2 Genital fold	8 Dorsal tendinous part of the urethral muscle
3 Bladder	
4 Right ureter	9 Fleshy part of the urethral muscle
5 Right ampulla of the deferent duct	10 Right lobe of the bulbourethral gland
6 Right vesicular gland (sometimes misleadingly called the seminal vesicle)	11 Bulb of the penis

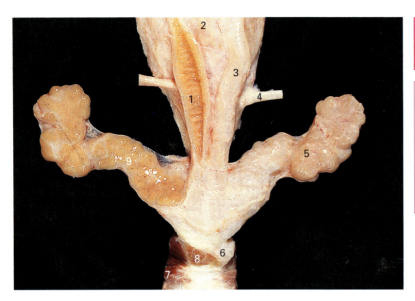

353. Detail of the neck of the bladder and the cranial part of the pelvic urethra in a bull with some of the male accessory glands opened.

1 Opened left ampulla showing the glandular mucosa
2 Neck of the bladder
3 Right ampulla
4 Right ureter
5 Right vesicular gland
6 Right half of the prostate body
7 Cranial extremity of the urethral muscle
8 Left half of the prostate body, sectioned close to the dorsal plane, to show its internal appearance
9 Left vesicular gland sectioned in the dorsal plane to show its internal appearance

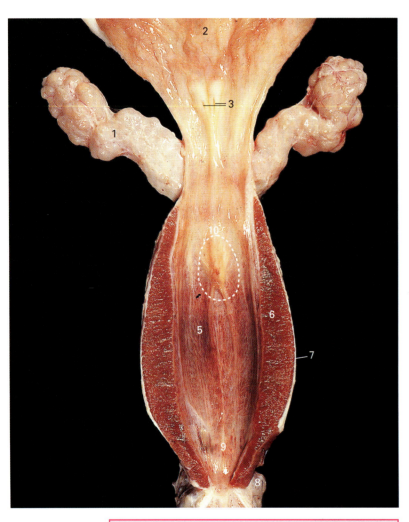

354. Bovine pelvic urethra opened from the ventral aspect.

1 Right vesicular gland
2 Mucosa of the bladder
3 Openings of the ureters
4 Left vesicular gland
5 Openings of the disseminate prostate glands
6 Urethral muscle
7 Fascia covering the urethral muscle
8 Left bulbourethral gland
9 Glandular openings
10 Colliculus seminalis where the openings of the ejaculatory ducts are located

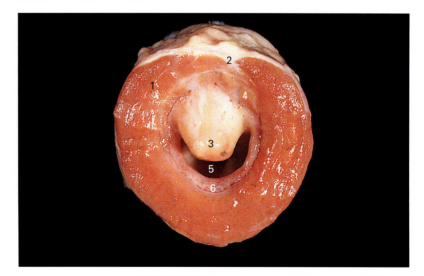

355. Caudal view of a transverse section of the pelvic urethra of a bull immediately caudal of the colliculus seminalis.

1 Fleshy part of the urethral muscle
2 Dorsal tendinous part of the urethral muscle
3 Colliculus seminalis
4 Disseminate part of the prostate gland
5 Urethral lumen
6 Spongy erectile tissue

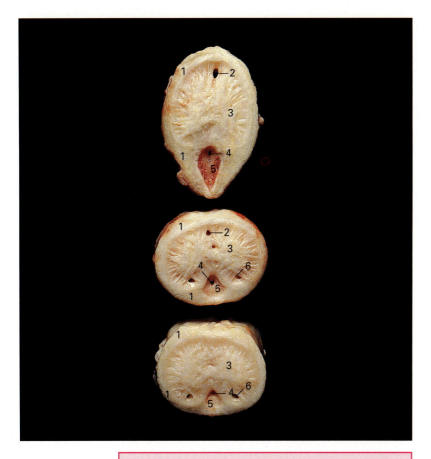

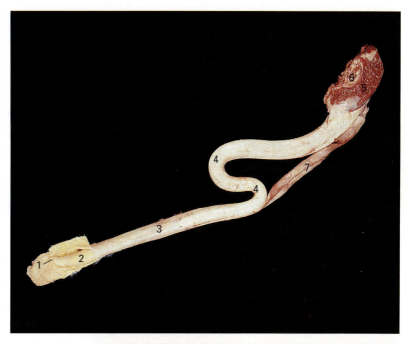

357. Left lateral view of the bovine penis.

1 Distal end of the penis	5 M. ischiocavernosus
2 Free mucosa-covered part of the body of the penis	6 Tunica albuginea surrounding the cavernous erectile tissue
3 Distal part of the body of the penis	7 M. retractor penis
4 Sigmoid flexure	

356. Transverse sections of the bovine penis from the proximal (top), middle (middle) and distal (bottom) parts of the shaft.

1 Tunica albuginea	4 Urethra
2 Dorsal vessel of the cavernous erectile tissue	5 Spongy erectile tissue (corpus spongiosum)
3 Cavernous erectile tissue (corpus cavernosum)	6 Ventrolateral vessels of the cavernous erectile tissue

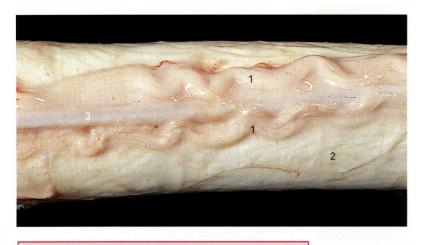

358. Detail of the dorsal surface of the bovine penis

1 Dorsal nerves	3 Dorsal artery
2 Tunica albuginea	

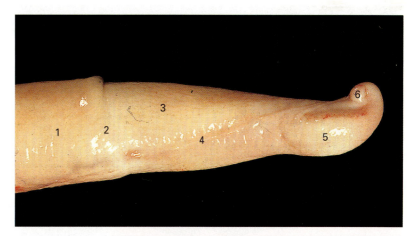

359. Right lateral view of the distal end of the bovine penis.

1 Reflected mucous lining of the prepuce	4 Raphe
2 Line of mucosal reflection	5 Glans
3 Mucosa covering the free part of the penile body	6 Urethral process

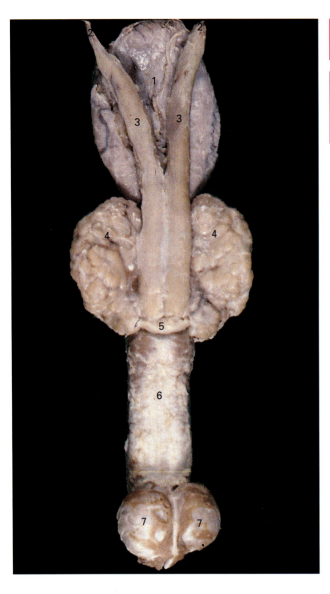

360. Dorsal view of the male accessory glands of a ram: formalin fixed specimen.

1 Bladder
2 Deferent duct
3 Ampullae
4 Vesicular glands
5 Connective tissue band

6 Pelvic urethra showing the tendinous part of the urethral muscle on its dorsal surface
7 Bulbourethral glands

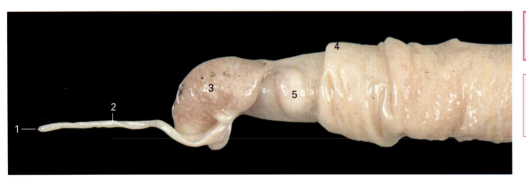

361. Distal part of the penis of a ram seen from the left. The areas of melanin pigmentation are normal in sheep.

1 Position of the urethral opening
2 Urethral process
3 Glans

4 Point of reflection of the prepuce; the prepuce has not been fully everted
5 Spongy tubercle

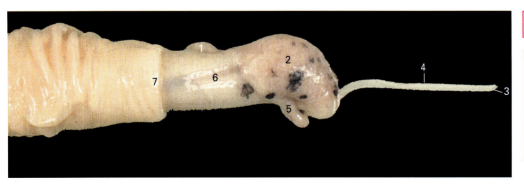

362. Distal part of the penis of a ram seen from the right.

1 Spongy tubercle
2 Glans
3 Position of the urethral opening
4 Urethral process
5 Proximal end of the urethral process

6 Course of the urethra and the surrounding spongy erectile tissue (corpus spongiosum) is shown by the oblique dark line
7 Point of reflection of the mucosa; the prepuce has not been fully everted

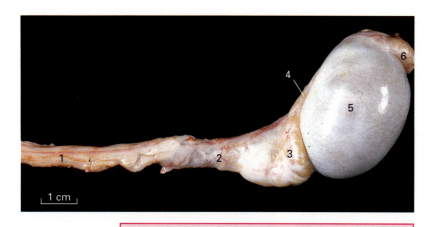

363. Lateral view of the left testis and related structures in a mature male llama

1 Spermatic cord	4 Body of the epididymis
2 Vascular cone of the testis	5 Lateral surface of the testis
3 Head of the epididymis	6 Tail of the epididymis

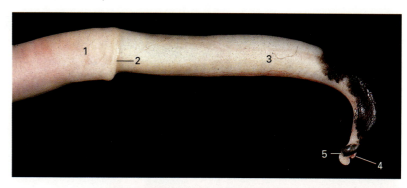

365. Left lateral view of the penis of a mature male llama. The areas of melanin pigmentation are normal.

1 Body of the penis covered by reflected preputial mucosa	3 Free part of the body of the penis
2 Line of reflection of the preputial mucosa	4 Tip of the urethral process
	5 Cartilaginous process

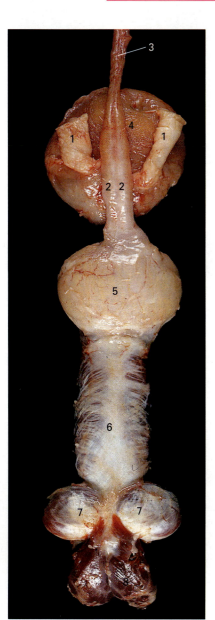

364. Dorsal view of the bladder, pelvic urethra and related structures in a mature male llama

1 Ureters
2 Ampullae of the deferent ducts
3 Deferent ducts
4 Bladder
5 Prostate
6 Pelvic urethra surrounded by the urethral muscle
7 Bulbourethral glands enclosed by skeletal muscle
8 Bulb of the penis

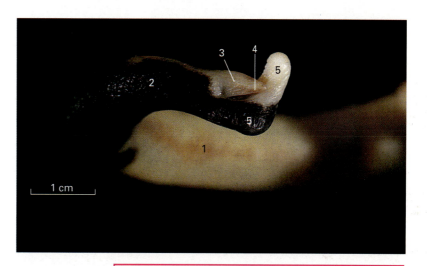

366. Detail of the distal end of the penis of a mature male llama

1 Free part of the body of the penis	3 Urethral process
2 Terminal part of the body of the penis	4 Position of the urethral opening
	5 Cartilagenous process

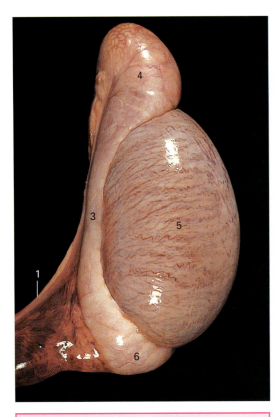

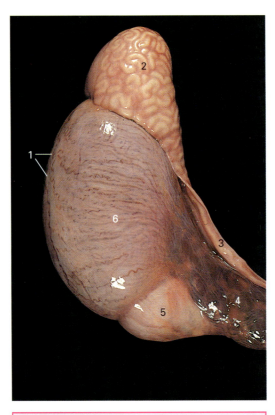

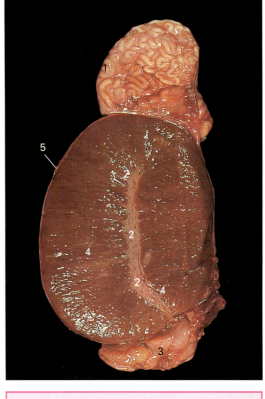

367. Lateral view of the left testis of a boar.

1 Deferent duct
2 Vascular cone of the testis
3 Body of the epididymis
4 Tail of the epididymis
5 Lateral surface of the testis showing the tortuous superficial branches of the testicular artery
6 Head of epididymis

368. Medial view of the left testis of a boar.

1 Free border of the testis
2 Tail of the epididymis
3 Deferent duct
4 Vascular cone of the testis
5 Head of the epididymis
6 Medial surface of the testis showing the tortuous superficial branches of the testicular artery

369. The testis of a boar sectioned in the sagittal plane.

1 Tail of the epididymis clearly showing the convolutions of the epididymal tubule
2 Mediastinum testis
3 Head of the epididymis
4 Small fibrous septa supporting the testicular parenchyma
5 Tunica albuginea

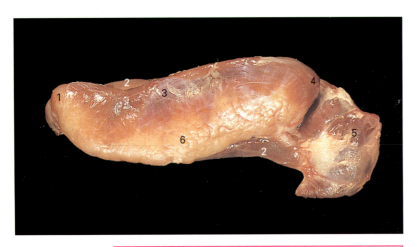

370. Lateral view of the bulbourethral glands and the penile bulb of a boar.

1 Cranial end of the left bulbourethral gland
2 Part of the pelvic urethra ensheathed in urethral muscle
3 Skeletal muscle covering the secretory tissue of the bulbourethral gland
4 Caudal end of the bulbourethral gland
5 M. bulbospongiosus
6 Secretory tissue of the bulbourethral gland seen through the fibrous sheath

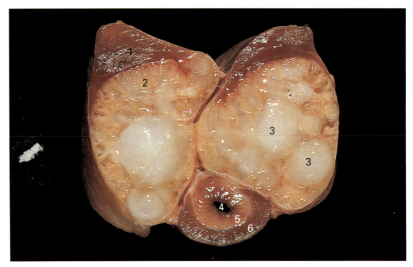

371. The bulbourethral glands and the pelvic urethra of a boar sectioned transversely at the midpoint of the glands.

1 Skeletal muscle on the dorsal aspect of the gland
2 Secretory tissue
3 Secretion
4 Pelvic urethra
5 Disseminate part of the prostate gland
6 Urethral muscle

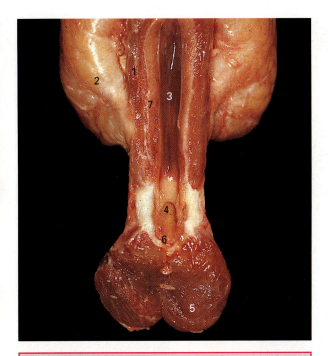

372. Ventral view of the caudal part of the pelvic urethra of a boar. The ventral side of the urethra has been removed to show the opening of the bulbourethral ducts.

1 Urethral muscle	5 Bulbospongiosus muscle
2 Secretory tissue of the bulbourethral gland	6 Cut edge of the urethral mucosa at the point where the urethra turns ventrally
3 Urethra	
4 Opening of the bulbourethral ducts	7 Disseminate part of the prostate gland

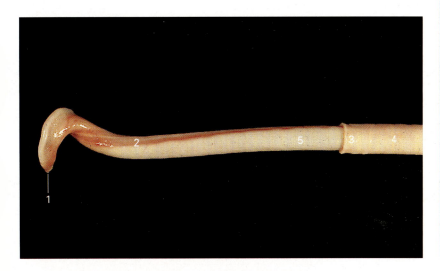

373. The distal extremity of the penis of a boar seen from the right side.

1 Position of the urethral orifice	3 Reflection of the preputial mucosa
2 Course of the urethra and the surrounding spongy erectile tissue (corpus spongiosum) is shown by the reddish line	4 Reflected parietal layer of the preputial mucosa
	5 Body of the penis

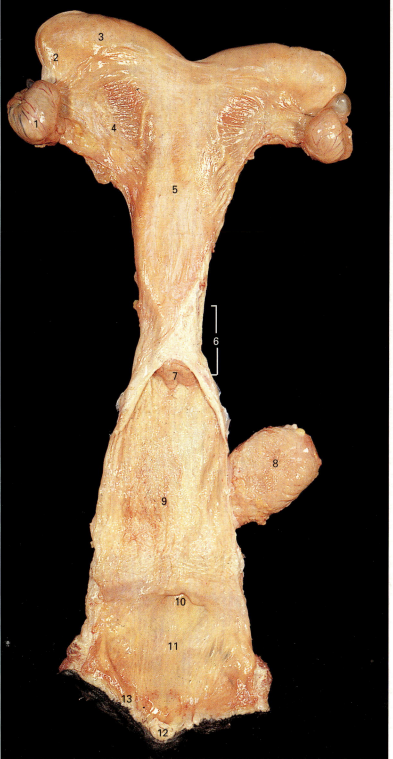

374. Dorsal view of the reproductive tract of a mare. The vagina and vestibule have been opened from the dorsal side.

1 Ovary	8 Bladder
2 Tip of the left uterine horn	9 Vagina
3 Left uterine horn	10 Urethral opening
4 Broad ligament	11 Vestibule
5 Body of the uterus	12 Clitoris
6 Position of the cervix	13 Vulva
7 External opening of the cervix	

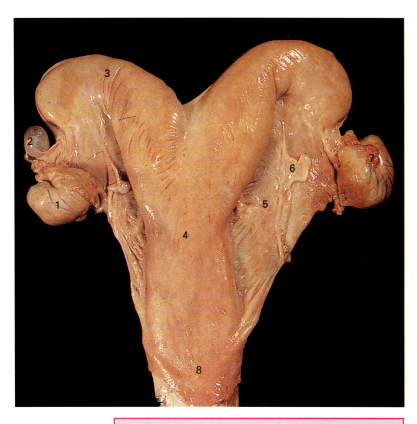

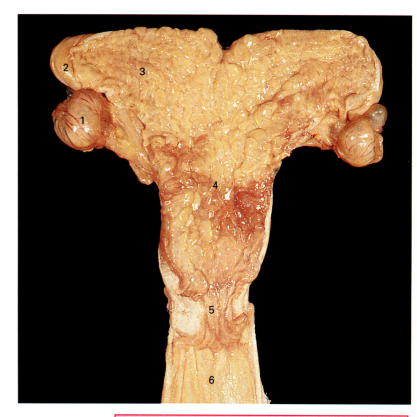

375. Ventral view of the uterus and related structures in the mare.

1 Ovary	5 Broad ligament
2 Para-ovarian cyst, a common and innocuous abnormality	6 Round ligament of the uterus
	7 Fimbria of the uterine tube (oviduct)
3 Right horn of the uterus	8 Position of the cervix
4 Body of the uterus	

376. Dorsal view of the uterus and related structures in the mare opened from the dorsal side.

1 Ovary	4 Mucosa of the body of the uterus
2 Tip of the left uterine horn	5 Cervix
3 Mucosa of the left uterine horn	6 Vagina

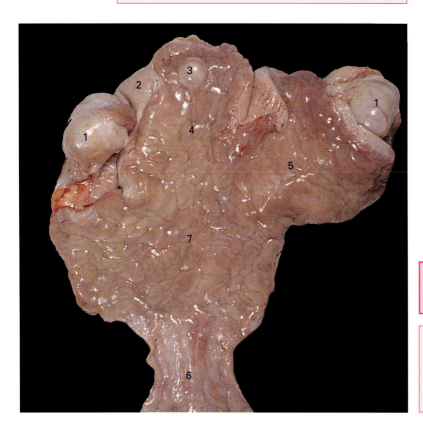

377. Dorsal view of the uterus of a pregnant mare 13 days after ovulation. It has been opened from the dorsal side.

1 Ovaries	4 Base of the left uterine horn
2 Unopened part of the left uterine horn	5 Base of the right uterine horn
3 Embryo lying on the endometrium (2 cm in diameter)	6 Cervix
	7 Body of the uterus

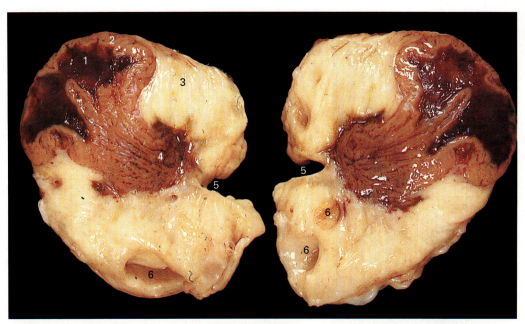

378. An equine ovary sectioned from the convex mesovarial border to the free concave border bearing the ovarian fossa. The cut surfaces of both halves are shown.

1 Central clot in a recently formed corpus luteum
2 Luteal tissue
3 Interstitial tissue of the ovary
4 Tongue of luteal tissue extending towards the ovarian fossa indicating the route followed at ovulation
5 Ovarian fossa (ovulation fossa)
6 Small ovarian follicles

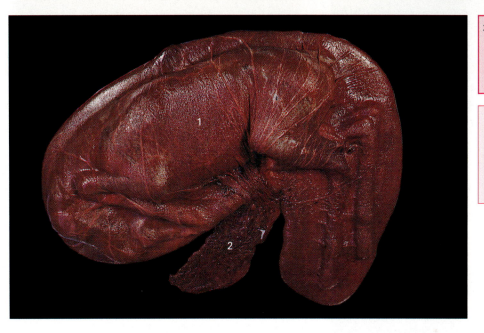

379. The conceptus of a mare removed from the uterus. All that can be seen directly is the exterior of the allantochorion. The allantochorion has the diffuse, microcotyledonary form that is characteristic of equids. Ten months' gestation.

1 Principal part of the allantochorion containing the fetus; it occupied the body of the uterus and the uterine horn in which fixation of the embryo occurred
2 Smaller part of the allantochorion that occupied the other uterine horn

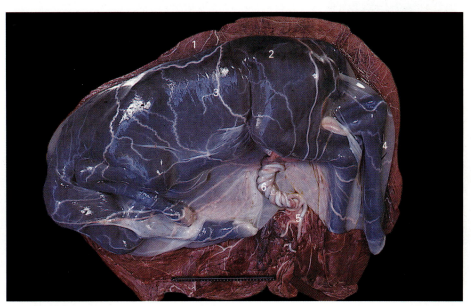

380. The same specimen as that seen in the previous photograph. The allantochorion has been opened to show the fetus lying within the amnion (scale = 30 cm).

1 Allantochorion
2 Amnion
3 Branches of the allantoic vessels supplying the amnion
4 Part of the amnion containing amniotic fluid
5 Allantoic vessels ramifying on the inner surface of the allantochorion
6 Allantoic part of the umbilical cord

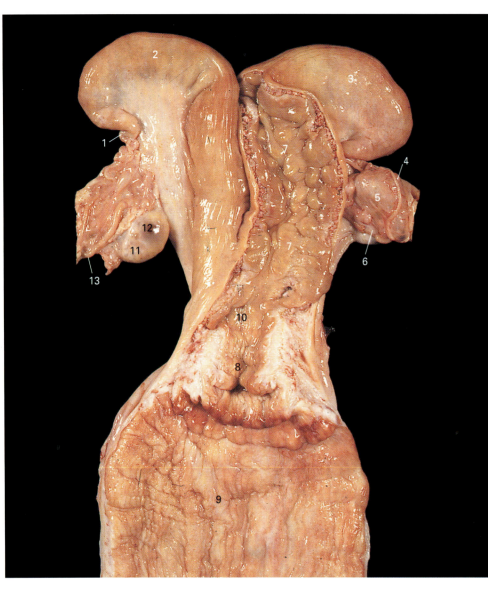

381. Dorsal view of the reproductive tract of a parous cow.
The cranial part of the vagina, the cervix, the body of the
uterus and part of the right horn have been opened from
the dorsal side.

1 Uterotubal junction
2 Left horn of the uterus
3 Right horn of the uterus
4 Isthmus of the uterine tube
  (oviduct)
5 Right ovary enveloped in the
  ovarian bursa; the uterine
  tube runs in the wall of the
  bursa
6 Ampulla of the uterine tube
  (oviduct)

7 Opened part of the right
  uterine horn; the mucosal
  projections are caruncles
8 Cervix
9 Cranial part of the vagina
10 Body of the uterus
11 Left ovary
12 Large ovarian follicle
13 Left uterine tube
  (oviduct)

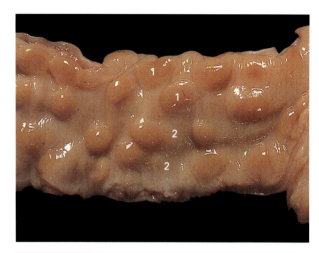

382. The middle part of the uterine horn of a
non-pregnant cow opened to show the mucosa.

1 Caruncles   2 Intercaruncular areas

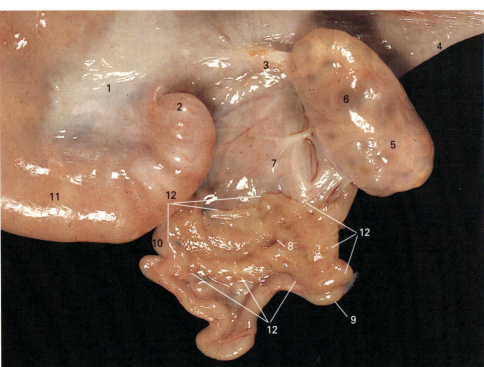

383. The ovary and associated structures in a cow. Note that
mesometrium, mesosalpinx and mesovarium can only
be imprecisely delineated but form parts of a functional
unit that can conveniently be referred
to as the broad ligament.

1 Mesometrium
2 Tip of the uterine horn;
  because the extreme end of
  the uterus is turned away
  from the camera, the
  uterotubal junction cannot
  be seen
3 Mesovarium
4 Cut edge of the
  mesometrium

5 Ovary
6 Medium sized follicle
7 Mesosalpinx
8 Infundibular opening
9 Ampulla of the uterine tube
  (oviduct)
10 Isthmus of the uterine
  tube (oviduct)
11 Uterine horn
12 Outline of the fimbria

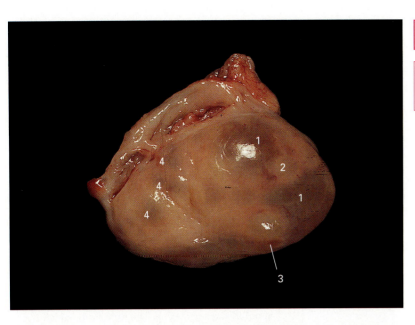

384. Bovine ovary containing a large follicle.

1 Preovulatory follicle	3 Luteal scar
2 Small antral follicles overlying the larger one	4 Numerous small antral follicles

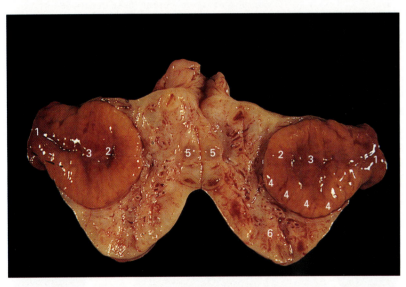

385. A bovine ovary sectioned longitudinally from the free border towards the attachment of the mesovarium. The cut surfaces face the camera and show an active corpus luteum during the early luteal phase (scale = 1 cm).

1 Part of the corpus luteum that protrudes from the ovarian surface at the point of ovulation	3 Residue of the central blood clot often formed at the time of ovulation
2 Part of the corpus luteum buried within other ovarian tissues	4 Fully developed luteal tissue
	5 Small ovarian follicles
	6 Interstitial tissue

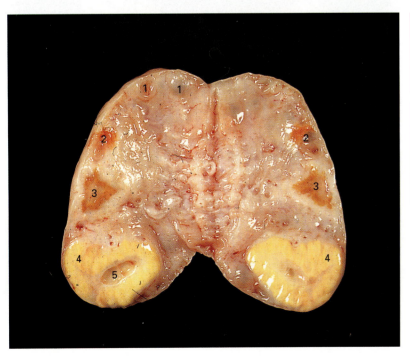

386. A bovine ovary sectioned longitudinally from the free border towards the attachment of the mesovarium. It has been opened so that both cut surfaces face the camera and shows corpora lutea of the oestrous cycle in various stages of regression.

1 Small follicles	4 Corpus luteum that has only recently begun to regress
2 Remnants of the corpus luteum of the antepenultimate cycle	
3 Remnants of the corpus luteum of the penultimate cycle	5 Small central cavity in the corpus luteum; this is not always present but is not abnormal

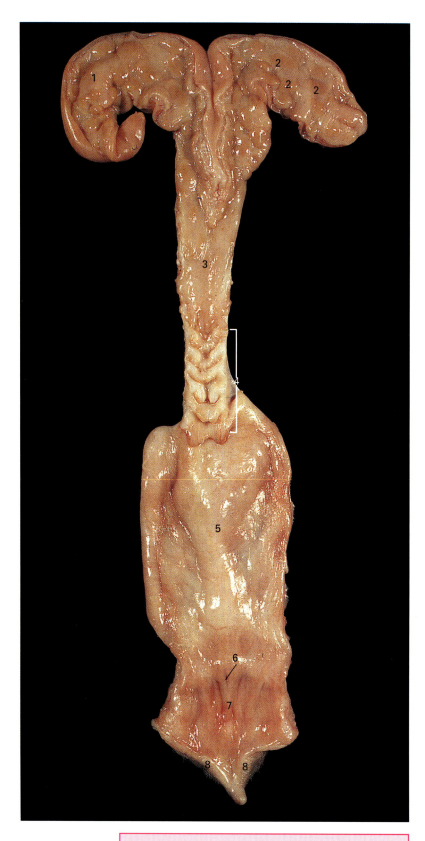

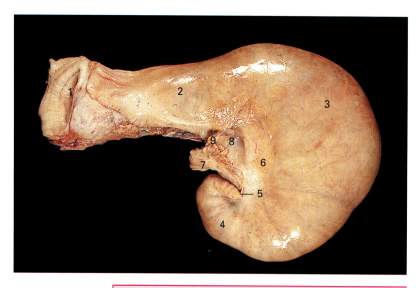

387. Lateral view of the pregnant uterus of a cow at about 80 days gestation. The right horn, which contains the fetus, entirely obscures the left horn.

1 Vaginal opening of the cervix
2 Body of the uterus
3 Middle part of the uterine horn containing the fetus
4 Tip of the uterine horn containing allantochorion only
5 Uterotubal junction
6 Broad ligament of the uterus (mesometrium, mesosalpinx and mesovarium)
7 Cut attachment of the more caudal part of the broad ligament
8 Ovary containing the corpus luteum of pregnancy
9 Ampulla of the uterine tube (oviduct)

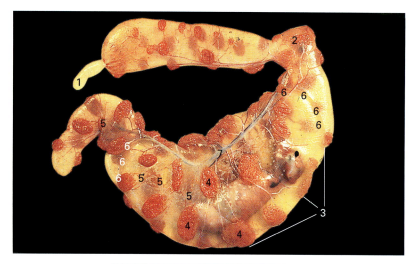

388. A bovine conceptus carefully separated from the endometrium. About 100 days' gestation.

1 Necrotic tip at the end of the arm of the allantochorion occupying the horn of the uterus that does not contain the fetus
2 Part of the allantochorion lying in the body of the uterus
3 Part of the allantochorion occupying the horn of the uterus that contains the fetus
4 Cotyledons
5 Intercotyledonary area
6 Limit of the amnion
7 Axial placental blood vessels

389. The tubular genitalia of a ewe opened from the dorsal side. The ovaries have been removed.

1 Left uterine horn
2 Typical caruncles, in this case forming part of the endometrium of the right horn
3 Body of the uterus
4 Cervix
5 Vagina
6 External urethral opening
7 Vestibule
8 Vulva

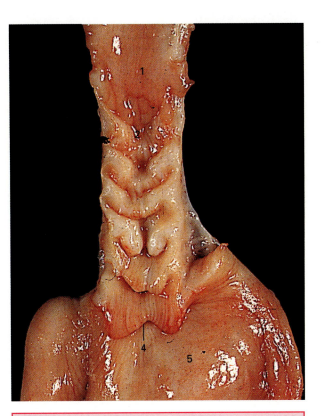

390. Detail of the cervix of a ewe.

1 Endometrium	canal is seen in dorsal
2 Internal opening	section at this level
3 One of the circular folds of	4 External opening
the cervix; the cervical	5 Vaginal mucosa

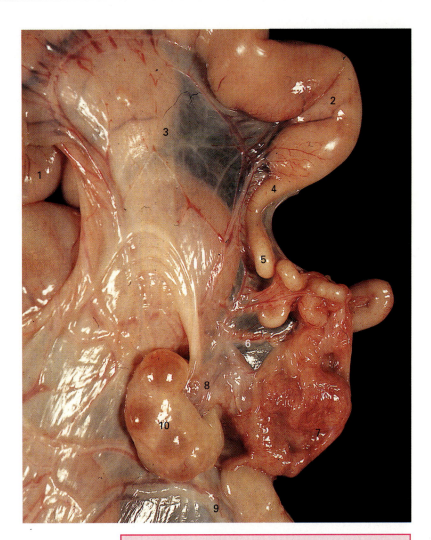

391. The right ovary and related structures in a ewe.

1 Middle of the right uterine horn	6 Mesosalpinx
2 Tip of the right uterine horn	7 Fimbria of the uterine tube
3 Mesometrium	8 Mesovarium
4 Uterotubal junction	9 Uterine artery
5 Isthmus of the uterine tube (oviduct)	10 Ovary containing four large follicles

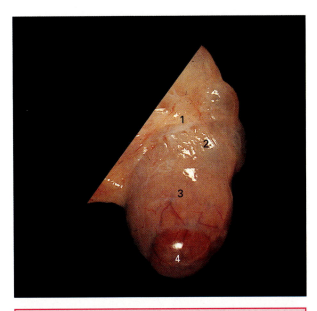

392. The ovary of a sheep containing a recently formed corpus luteum.

1 Mesovarium	4 Small amount of luteal
2 Ovary	tissue protruding from the
3 Large swelling within the	ovarian surface at the site
ovary indicates the	of ovulation
position of most of the	
luteal tissue	

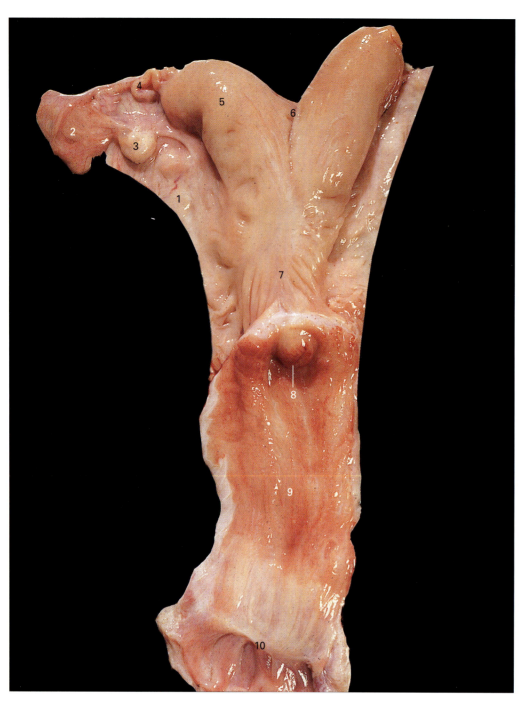

393. Dorsal view of the female reproductive tract of a llama. The vagina has been opened from the dorsal side. The right ovary and most of the vestibule have been removed.

1	Broad ligament of the uterus	6	Intercornual ligament
2	Fimbria	7	Body of the uterus
3	Ovary	8	External opening of the cervix
4	Isthmus of the uterine tube (oviduct)	9	Vagina
5	Left uterine horn	10	Junction of the vagina and vestibule

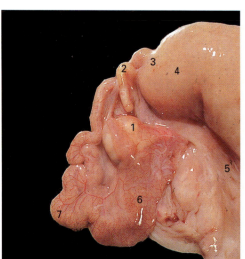

394. The tip of the left uterine horn and related structures in a llama.

1	Left ovary enveloped by the wall of the ovarian bursa (the free part of the mesosalpinx)	4	Tip of the left uterine horn
		5	Broad ligament of the uterus
2	Isthmus of the uterine tube (oviduct)	6	Fimbria
3	Uterotubal junction	7	Ampulla of the uterine tube (oviduct)

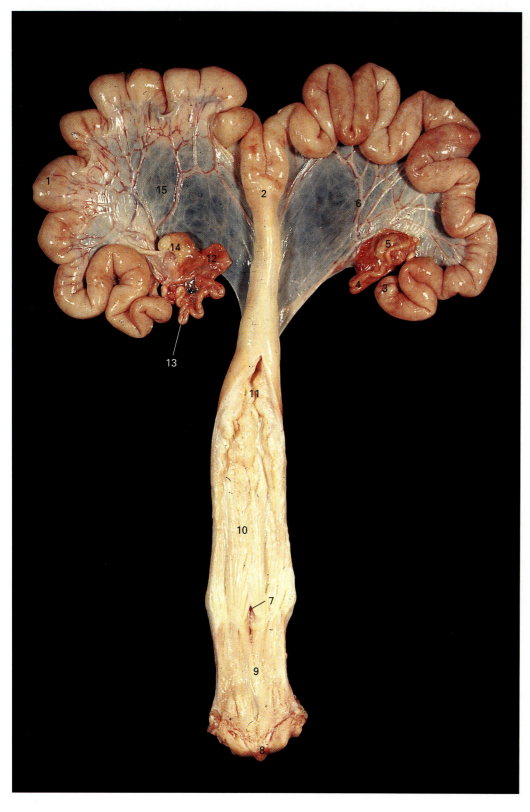

395. Dorsal view of the female reproductive tract of a pig. The vagina and vestibule have been opened from the dorsal side.

1 Left uterine horn
2 Body of the uterus
3 Tip of the right uterine horn
4 Right uterine tube (oviduct)
5 Right ovary enveloped by the wall of the ovarian bursa (the free part of the mesosalpinx)
6 Branches of the uterine artery and the utero-ovarian vein
7 Urethral opening
8 Vulva
9 Vestibule
10 Vagina
11 Vaginal opening of the cervix showing some of the more caudal interlocking tubercles (pulvini)
12 Fimbria of the uterine tube
13 Left uterine tube (oviduct)
14 Left ovary exposed following retraction of the ovarian bursa
15 Broad ligament of the uterus

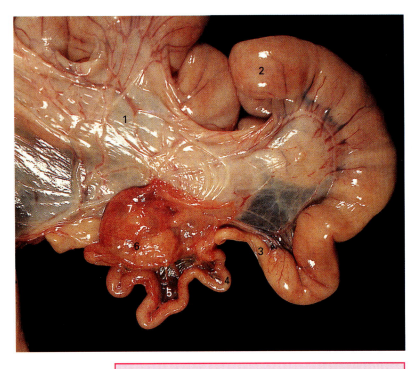

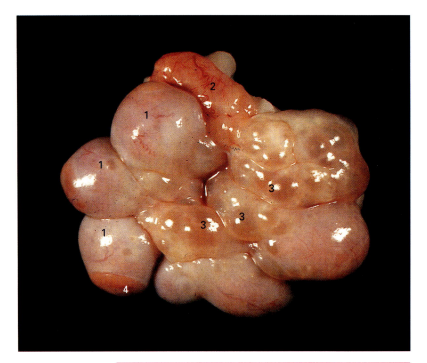

396. Detail of the uterine tube (oviduct) and related structures in a pig.

1 Broad ligament of the uterus
2 Right uterine horn
3 Uterotubal junction
4 Isthmus of the uterine tube
5 Mesosalpinx
6 Ovary seen through the free part of the mesosalpinx
7 Fimbria of the uterine tube

397. The ovary of a pig.

1 Corpora lutea
2 Cut mesovarium
3 Medium sized ovarian follicles
4 Luteal tissue protruding through the point of ovulation

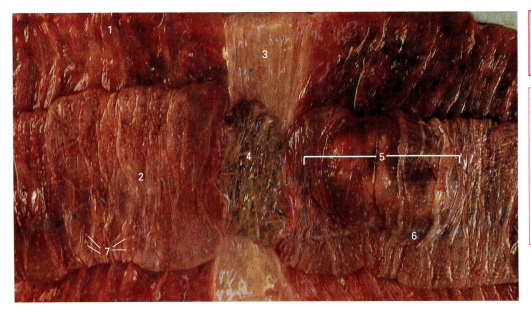

398. The placenta of a pig. The specimen shows a short section of the uterus opened along the mesometrial side to reveal parts of two conceptuses lying on the endometrium. About 42 days' gestation.

1 Highly vascularized placental part of the endometrium
2 Part of the allantochorion of the conceptus to the left dilated by allantoic fluid
3 Poorly vascularized interlocular part of the endometrium
4 Entangled necrotic tips of the conceptuses to the right and left
5 Amnion of the conceptus on the right, containing the fetus surrounded by amniotic fluid
6 Primary branches of the placental vessels visible through the allantochorion
7 Regular areolae